# Newborn Beauty

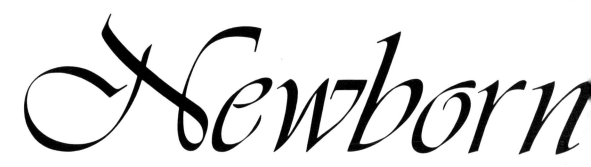

# Newborn

A·COMPLETE·BEAUTY, HEALTH
TO THE NINE MONTHS
AND THE NINE

*by Wende Devlin Gates and*

WITH A PREFACE BY
PHOTOGRAPHS BY MICHAEL PATEMAN

# Beauty

## AND ENERGY GUIDE
## OF PREGNANCY
## MONTHS AFTER

### Gail McFarland Meckel

GIDEON G. PANTER, M.D.
ILLUSTRATIONS BY DURELL GODFREY

THE VIKING PRESS • NEW YORK

LIBRARY OF CONGRESS CATALOGING IN PUBLICATION DATA
Gates, Wende.
  Newborn beauty.
  Includes index.
  1. Pregnancy.  2. Prenatal care.  3. Postnatal
care.  4. Beauty, Personal.  I. Meckel, Gail, joint
author.  II. Title.
RG525.G36    618.2'4    79-56263
ISBN 0-670-57310-8

Printed in the United States of America
Set in CRT Garamond

DESIGNED BY BETH TONDREAU
WITH ASSISTANCE FROM SHAREN DUGOFF

For my children,
Christopher and Bryan,
with love
W.D.G.


For Bill, Alexandra,
and Mother,
who mean so much to me
G.M.M.

# Preface

PREGNANCY is usually one of the most carefully planned events in our lives. Even when pregnancy is unplanned, most of us began anticipating it in early childhood: playing "house" is a universal game of childhood. In all cultures little boys take their turns as "father" to little girls being "mother," and the part of the baby is played by a doll, or a younger sibling, or even the family dog.

In spite of this kind of play practice during childhood, and in spite of thought and study and preparation for parenting during early adulthood, we must all deal with many ambivalent feelings when pregnancy finally occurs. And these insecure feelings recur, although to a lesser degree, with each pregnancy.

The feelings have to do with general psychological concepts and with practical physical issues. You wonder, Will I be a good parent? Will my husband love the baby? And other insecure feelings occur. Will my husband love me when I'm pregnant? Will he still think that I'm attractive? How can I keep myself looking good? What will happen to my body?

Because pregnancy is a time of heightened feelings, pregnant women are often especially confused and distracted by the bodily changes that take place. And the pregnant mother hesitates to ask her doctor any but the most serious of the many questions that go through her mind every day of the pregnancy.

The changing hormones cause skin and hair changes. There are issues of diet and weight gain. There are mechanical problems due to the increasing uterine size, with its accompanying pressure changes. And varicose veins, and moles, and skin growths. And all these transformations are occurring at a time when the new parents-to-be are still dealing with their sometimes conflicting feelings.

Wende Gates and Gail Meckel have written a book that gives the pregnant woman sensible practical advice about her everyday bodily concerns, and have richly illustrated it with first-person accounts with which every pregnant woman can identify. There are interesting, safe formulas for skin cleansers and creams. The book has prudent nutritional advice and sample diets. There are exercises, explanations of common medical problems, advice on makeup and styles of dress, and tips on how to deal with day-to-day body changes.

Although pregnant women may be reluctant to ask their obstetricians about how pregnancy affects their looks and feelings, questions about quasi-medical issues, pregnancy-related beauty problems, and even—in some cases—"frivolous" matters are not irrelevant. *Newborn Beauty: A Complete Beauty, Health, and Energy Guide to the Nine Months of Pregnancy and the Nine Months After* answers these questions. It gives the pregnant woman the kind of information she seeks, without having to justify its medical importance. And there is no doubt that someone who looks good will usually feel better as a result.

GIDEON G. PANTER, M.D.

# Acknowledgments

WHILE WRITING THIS BOOK we sought help from experts in many fields, as well as from friends and colleagues. We want to express our gratitude to those men and women who shared with us their knowledge, talent, and in particular their time, to help create *Newborn Beauty*.

At the beginning we wish to thank the many medical experts who shared their valuable information and time with us. They are: Howard T. Bellin, M.D., Assistant Professor of Plastic Surgery, New York Medical College, Chief of Plastic Surgery, Cabrini Medical Center, New York City; Marvin W. Bromberg, D.D.S.; Steven Clarke, Ph.D., Assistant Professor of Nutrition, Ohio State University; Harry Condrea, M.D., Clinical Assistant Professor of Obstetrics and Gynecology, New York Medical College, Assistant Attending Obstetrician and Gynecologist, Beth Israel Hospital, Chief of Gynecology, Medical Arts Center Hospital, New York City; Charles P. DeFeo, M.D., Clinical Professor of Dermatology, New York University Hospital, Attending Dermatologist, Lenox Hill Hospital, and Chief of Service, Saint Clare's Hospital; Sandra Haber, Ph.D., Director of Psychological Services, Howard M. Shapiro Medical Association; Bonnie Jacobson, Ph.D., Associate Director, Park East Psychological Associates and Growth Skills; Fritzi Kallop, Assistant Clinical Nurse Specialist and Lamaze Instructor, New York Hospital; Sherwin A. Kaufman, M.D., P.C., Associate

Attending Obstetrician and Gynecologist, Lenox Hill Hospital, New York City; Mary Ellen Keaveny, Associate Professor of Maternal and Child Health, College of Staten Island; Irwin I. Lubowe, M.D., Clinical Professor of Dermatology Emeritus, New York Medical College; Norman Orentreich, M.D., Clinical Associate Professor of Dermatology, New York University School of Medicine; Pedro Rosso, M.D., Associate Professor of Pediatrics, Columbia University; Robert G. Schwager, M.D., Attending Plastic Surgeon, New York Hospital, Assistant Professor of Surgery, Cornell University Medical College; Maria Day Simonson, Sc.D., Ph.D., Assistant Professor, Johns Hopkins Institutions, and Director of the Health and Weight Program, Department of Psychiatry; Don Sloan, M.D., Assistant Professor of Obstetrics and Gynecology and Director of Psychosomatics, New York Medical College, Lenox Hill Hospital; Alan G. Snart, M.D., Assistant Professor of Medicine, Cornell University Medical School; Carol Diamond Taney, M.S., Psychologist; Esther Wallace, B.S., R.D., Director of the New York Hospital Clinic of Nutrition; Murray Weisenfeld, Doctor of Podiatric Medicine; Alvin C. Weseley, M.D., Associate Clinical Professor of Obstetrics and Gynecology, New York University School of Medicine.

Special thanks must be offered to Gideon G. Panter, M.D., Assistant Clinical Professor of Obstetrics and Gynecology at the New York Hospital-Cornell Medical Center, for his medical reading and friendly support over the three years it took to write this book. We are grateful to Alfred Tanz, M.D., Assistant Clinical Professor of Obstetrics and Gynecology, New York Medical College, Attending Obstetrician-Gynecologist, Lenox Hill Hospital, for making himself so accessible to answer our many questions. Dr. Hillard H. Pearlstein, M.D., Assistant Clinical Professor of Dermatology at the Mount Sinai School of Medicine of the City University of New York and the Mount Sinai Hospital, New York, read our chapters on skin and hair problems for medical accuracy. We're grateful to him for his time and kindness.

Many people at different nonprofit organizations provided invaluable information for this book, and we would like to thank them for that, and for the public service rendered by their organizations' research. We particularly want to express appreciation to Leslie Dach and Marcia Fine Silcox, Science Associates Environmental Defense Fund; the La Leche League; and the Cesarean Birth Association.

In the beauty, fashion, and exercise fields, the following experts shared their knowledge: Mario Badescu of Mario Badescu Skin Care Salon, New York City; Kenneth Battelle, Kenneth Beauty Salon; Kay Burgess, Maternity Manufacturer Representative; Philip Kingsley, trichologist, Philip Kingsley Trichological Center, New York and London; Georgette Klinger of Georgette Klinger Skin Care Salons; Judy Loeb, fashion designer and manufacturer; Didier Malige, freelance hairstylist; and Pierre Ouaknine of Pierre Michel Coiffures. We deeply appreciate their assistance. We would like to single out Pablo Manzoni, New York beauty expert, who offered support as well as his time and special talents. Diana Simkin, M.A., movement specialist and Lamaze prepared-childbirth instructor, created a special exercise program for our book and we are very grateful for her contribution and her guidance.

We were fortunate to work with photographer Michael Pateman. As a new father himself, he brought warmth and understanding of the subject to his pictures. As an artist, he has captured the beauty of pregnancy. We want to thank our illustrator, Durell Godfrey, who was a joy to work with. Her charm and wit are also reflected in her work.

We also want to extend affection and thanks to our families. From the beginning they gave us their unqualified support. We are grateful to Jeffrey A. Devlin and J. Charles Taney III, both of whom gave exceptional assistance for this book.

Of all the people we owe thanks to, the women we interviewed deserve the greatest praise. Their experiences, insights, and resourcefulness provide the essence of this book. We owe them a great deal. Susan Curtis deserves special acknowledgment for her help in conceiving this book and for her constant encouragement.

Lastly, love and thanks to our wonderful husbands, Geoffrey Gates and Bill Meckel. From their battle stations at the cribs, they urged us onward. Without them *Newborn Beauty* would not have been possible.

# Table of Contents

# Newborn Beauty

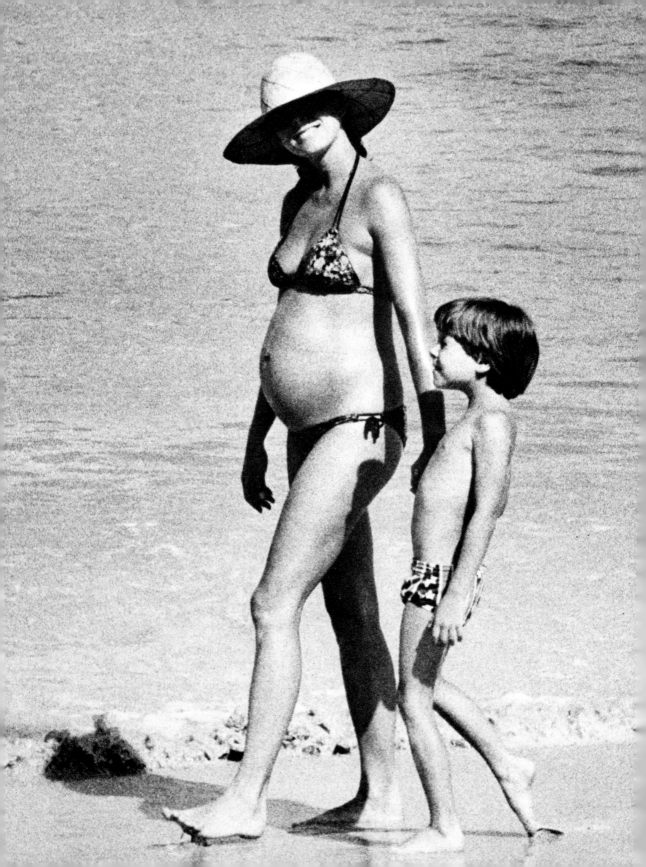

# *Introduction*

CONGRATULATIONS—you're pregnant! This new life growing within your body means the start of *your* new life—a new you who may feel sometimes elated, sometimes confused and uncertain. Many of your uncertainties revolve around your changing body. You're fascinated and perhaps fearful of the changes your looks will undergo. If you're at all like us you may have some of the questions we had.

"How can I stay looking chic and glamorous while I'm pregnant? I'm determined to look good these nine months."

"Can I prevent stretch marks?"

"Will jogging hurt the baby?"

"My husband likes me very slender. Will he be turned off by my bigness during pregnancy?"

"Can I lose the added weight of pregnancy quickly and still nurse?"

Your curiosity about how pregnancy will change your looks is not vanity. It's natural and justified. For as we are beginning to find out, pregnancy brings about changes not only in your waistline, but in your skin, hair, nails, posture, and sex life—to name a few. And the hormonal and physical changes of pregnancy can cause never-before encountered beauty problems: facial skin can darken in the sun; your hair may grow gloriously during pregnancy, then fall out after the baby's born; and your body can swell with water, giving you full lips, puffy eyes, and your whole face a slightly different look requiring new makeup tricks.

When we met in prepared-childbirth class in 1976, pregnant with our first babies, we were each working in the fashion and beauty magazine world and so we were perhaps more conscious of the way pregnancy affected our looks than we might otherwise have been. We discussed the idea of a pregnancy beauty book. But it was really when our friends asked us questions about how to take care of *their* pregnancy and new-mother problems that we knew there was a need for this kind of book. It would be dedicated to, and only to, the pregnant woman and new mother—not a book on the medical machinations of the body, but how pregnancy was going to affect our looks, bodies, health, sex lives, and energy.

We began interviewing women of all ages—pregnant women, new mothers, grandmothers, women we'd met through work, at the playground, or at a party, for their ideas about caring for themselves during the nine months of pregnancy and nine months after. The women we met loved sharing their ideas and pregnancy "street wisdom." Perhaps at no time is communication as open and intimate among women as during pregnancy and new motherhood. And this is the approach we used for this book—woman-to-woman.

This is not to mean we left out the experts. Doctors, nurses, nutritionists, hairdressers, cosmetologists all play key roles in *Newborn Beauty*. In fact, this book answers some of those questions you'd like to ask your obstetrician or dermatologist or internist, but feel he doesn't have the time for. For the most part doctors are not tuned into the cosmetic aspects of pregnancy. They are concerned with health and medical care and most of them don't stop to think that you might be worried by such "normal" pregnancy problems as spider veins or the discomforts of excess vaginal discharge, or that you might wonder if it's safe to color your hair during pregnancy. This book fills that void and answers all those beauty and health care questions you have at this time.

Reverence for pregnant women has been a primitive impulse that crops up in almost every culture and age. With fewer babies being born today, there seems to be a new pride in pregnancy—and this "pregnant and proud" attitude is important. If you feel you're looking your best, you will act and feel your best and people will respond to you accordingly. (And don't forget—now that you are pregnant, people will be scrutinizing you especially carefully!) If you think pregnancy is ugly, you are setting up a self-fulfilling prophecy.

The woman who emerges in this book is one whose self-image is strong during and after pregnancy. She and you are different from some of the pregnant women of yesterday. Women now work, entertain, jog, and enjoy sex right up to the end of pregnancy. They care for their bodies and make pregnancy glamorous instead of a burden. Even if you have to cope with some of the ills common to pregnancy, there's no reason to lose your excitement or self-confidence. One woman was nauseated and had headaches throughout the first trimester of her pregnancy. She also ended up gaining a lot more weight than she thought she would. She still thought she was the most beautiful pregnant woman ever. Your image of yourself and your positive attitude are paramount in helping you through these new problems. Fixing up the outside really does help fix up the inside!

One wonderful benefit of pregnancy is that it provides a clean slate. Since your baby will be affected by your health habits, you have to reconsider your diet (lunch is no longer a diet soda and taco but chicken breast and cottage cheese), how much sleep you get, how hard you work and play. The need to exercise suddenly takes on new meaning. Your sex life may delight or perplex you. You think about your wardrobe from a new point of view. If you were never particularly conscious of a beauty, health, and energy program before, pregnancy and its built-in changes force you to be so now. The positive changes you make now can last a lifetime!

We've written the pregnancy part of the book with the assumption that you'll have more time during pregnancy to spend on yourself than during the nine months after, especially if this is your first child. The beauty routines are streamlined in the "After" half of the book. Be mindful of the fact that your time is *very* limited when you have a new baby to care for and beauty care is obviously not the most important task in your life. Naturally you have other priorities. Practice your makeup and beauty care routines during your pregnancy so you'll be adept once the little one arrives. Go through your wardrobe with a critical eye towards what will work for your new life-style.

We strongly urge you to take prepared-childbirth classes. Even if you do not want to go through with natural childbirth, you will get a marvelous education in pregnancy and childbirth. You'll want to read other books about pregnancy, breast-feeding, childbirth and child-rearing, etc. This book won't answer all your questions. *Nor is it intended in any way to replace your doctor's professional advice.* Your doctor knows you and your particular medical problems better than anyone else so be sure to follow his or her instructions.

Most of the women photographed in this book are, or were, professional models and range in age from early twenties to late thirties. They were all pregnant (no pillows!) when their pictures were taken for the first half of this book and all had beautiful babies. Their life-styles are varied. One goes to acting class. Another goes to art school. One is a teacher and one is an accomplished artist. Since modeling is a profession for most of them, they must stay in shape and look beautiful all the time. As models in fashion magazines do, we thought these women and their beauty would inspire all of us to care for ourselves and look our best as well. They had their problems too—but knew how to take care of them when they occurred.

Writing this book has been thrilling for us. Following the pregnancies of the many women we interviewed to the birth of their babies and after gave us a chance to relive the incredible joy and pleasure pregnancy, birth, and motherhood bring.

Have a happy and beautiful pregnancy!

# CHAPTER·1·
## All About Skin During Pregnancy

"YOUR SKIN IS BLOOMING," someone says to you. "You're really one of those beautiful, glowing pregnant women." And of course you *are* beautiful. You're six months pregnant and your skin is smooth, rosy, and supple as a result of the changes pregnancy brings about in your body—changes that often give pregnant women the most beautiful skin they've had in their lives.

For all the billions of dollars spent in the cosmetic and dermatology business, experts still haven't found a way to copy the process that brings about the beautiful effects of pregnancy. While you lose your waistline, chances are that you will also lose your pimples or acne since excess estrogen produced by the placenta slows the flow of sebum in the oil glands. Your skin clears up—often for good. And the increased supply of estrogen makes the blood vessels close to the surface of your skin dilate, which gives you your rosy glow.

*All* is not rosy, however; the changes of pregnancy can also cause skin problems such as spider veins, stretch marks, dry or oily skin, acne, itching, and skin discoloration. And you may have questions like the ones some of our friends asked us:

"How can I prevent stretch marks?"

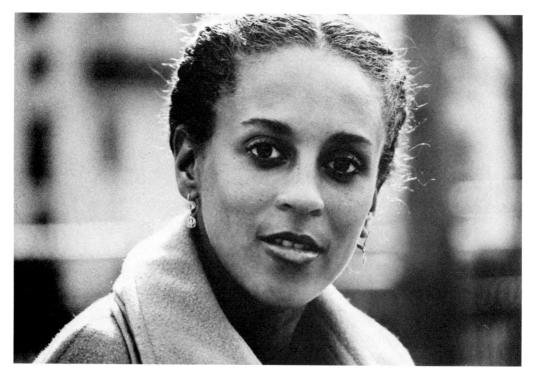

Alva's skin exudes the health and glow that pregnancy often brings.

"What are these red, spidery outbursts on my cheeks? Will they disappear?"

"What's this brown line up my stomach and will it go away after I have my baby?"

"What happens when you tan a pregnant stomach?"

"I have to have a Caesarean section delivery. What will the scar look like?"

"My doctor wants me to stop taking baths and start taking showers during my last two months of pregnancy. Why?"

"My face looks heavier and puffier in this last trimester. What kind of makeup can I use to make my eyes look less puffy?"

"I feel like I'm piling on more and more makeup since I've been pregnant. Maybe I'm compensating for looking so heavy. I need a whole new look—any suggestions?"

Some of these questions will already have occurred to you; others may never come up; and there are still others we haven't asked here. But in this chapter we'll try to cover all the problems as well as the benefits of pregnancy when it comes to beautiful skin. That way you'll know what the problems are and how to deal with them—though you should never seek to correct them without medical supervision. One pregnant friend of ours ran to an expensive electrolysis center to have three spider veins removed with an electric needle, not realizing that ninety percent of spider veins or spider angiomas (which are very common in pregnancy), disappear or recede within three months after the baby is born. If she had consulted her doctor he would have told her this; as it was, the holes caused by the electric needle (and the hole in her pocket) remained.

Whatever happens to your skin during pregnancy, remember the watchword is "wait." Within six months after giving birth, ninety percent of *all* your skin changes—including, alas, the rosy glow—disappear as surprisingly as they appeared.

## WHAT CAUSES SKIN CHANGES DURING PREGNANCY?

HORMONES, HORMONES, HORMONES. Most changes in the skin result from the tremendous increase in hormones in your pretty pregnant body. When you aren't pregnant your skin's beauty and health are affected by only two hormone producers: the ovaries and the adrenal gland. Pregnancy introduces your body to a new worker: the placenta and fetus, or the "feto-placental unit."

It takes a good two to three months after conception for the feto-placental unit to start producing its own set of hormones in significant amounts. When it does, it jolts your system with new supplies of estrogen, progesterone, and sixteen to eighteen other hormones, many of which are appearing for the first time in your life. Although scientists don't know exactly how your hormones fluctuate during pregnancy and lactation to affect the condition of your skin, they do know that similar endocrine upheavals occur during adolescence and menopause, as well as during periods of emotional stress and sickness.

GENES, GENES, GENES. Jan and Linda may have similar hormone levels. They may experience the same amount of stress and they may rest and eat exactly alike. But only Linda will get oily skin and pimples while she's pregnant. Why? Linda has a higher "end organ sensitivity" inherited from her parents. The "end organ" involved here is the oil glands. Linda's oil glands are more sensitive to the new hormone levels in the blood stream and begin to produce more oil. Jan's sebaceous glands are resistant and her skin looks clear and rosy.

Almost all skin changes of pregnancy, including stretch marks, spider veins, acne, etc., are caused by hormonal changes and your body's genetic susceptibility to these new hormone levels. Years ago when *you* were being conceived, you received a genetic code which spelled out a lifetime program for the condition of your skin, including end organ sensitivity. Whether we like it or not, great skin usually comes from great genes. Good care of your skin is enormously important, but genes rank first.

Ask your mother what happened to her skin during her pregnancy. Ask your father about his skin at your age. Not all skin changes may be brought about by pregnancy. They can occur at any age and may simply coincide with these nine months. But we can be thankful that dermatologists now know much more than when your mother was pregnant. No one has to suffer from a bad skin condition.

## WHAT IS GOING TO HAPPEN TO MY SKIN?
## PROBLEMS AND SOLUTIONS

You needn't allow the joys of expecting a baby to be haunted by fears of stretch marks and other skin changes. Of course we've all heard the horror stories about the physical changes of pregnancy. And although we know we can always lose the weight gained during pregnancy, skin changes—especially permanent ones—are particularly distressing. After all, our skin is all that stands between ourselves and the world. But being armed with the facts of each particular problem should help remove some of the fearful mystique. The following section details all the skin problems of pregnancy. If your skin problems are serious, consult a dermatologist—who, in turn, should be in touch with your obstetrician.

STRETCH MARKS. Barbara started noticing slight reddish streaks on her abdomen in her seventh month of pregnancy. She'd heard about stretch marks and wondered if that's what these streaks were. Her doctor told her they were—and that nothing could be done about them. Her skin was simply not elastic enough to bear the weight of the baby. "You're having a baby," he said, "and it's not easy on your skin. Unfortunately stretch marks are one of the prices women pay. Try to be philosophical."

Try as she could, Barbara could not be philosophical. She was very upset. "I'm not a model or a movie star," she said in a sad voice. "But I still want to be able to wear a bikini. I want to look good—for my husband, and most of all for me. I want my old body back—I don't want to have scars!"

After Barbara's baby was born, she found the stretch marks shrank considerably. She could wear a bikini—and getting a tan did wonders in masking the marks. "I'll never be *happy* about my stretch marks," she said a year after the baby was born. "But I *am* more philosophical now. They don't bother me as much as I thought they would and my husband says he couldn't care less. Somehow, stretch marks seem like a small price to pay for being a mother and having my little boy."

It is never easy to accept bodily scarring, even if you share Barbara's feelings about the rewards. Reactions to stretch marks are obviously varied; some women find severe, plainly visible stretch marks unbearably ugly and turn to plastic surgeons for help. But our interviews found that most women who get stretch marks—and reports show that fifty percent of all pregnant women do—are not overly concerned. Look over your body carefully right now: you probably have some stretch marks on your hips, buttocks, thighs, or breasts already. Almost all women and most men get stretch marks when their bodies grow and change rapidly during adolescence.

Stretch marks may begin as early as the first month of pregnancy. They first appear as slightly depressed reddish or brownish streaks on the skin of the abdomen, buttocks, hips, thighs, and breasts of the pregnant woman. After delivery they become flat, silvery-whitish streaks. Scientists argue about how stretch marks occur. Some say the increased hormonal output associated with pregnancy (or adolescence) tends to weaken the collagen, a type of protein found in connective tissue, which is the supporting structure of the skin. The elastic tissues are permanently traumatized by sudden growth, and scarring occurs. Others say the swelling of the abdomen and breasts, plus the added weight of pregnancy, actually stretches the skin. It seems reasonable to suppose that both these points of view have merit: your skin, already weakened by the increased fragility of the collagen, may indeed be stretched to its limit by your pregnancy. Whether you get stretch marks or not is probably genetically determined. Your "end organs"—the collagen here—may or may not be resistant to the new hormone levels. One woman we know gained seventy pounds and didn't develop one stretch mark; another gained twenty and developed a bunch. Although the skin of black women is not more susceptible to stretch marks than that of white women, stretch marks are more apparent.

Whatever their cause, once you get them, stretch marks are discouragingly difficult to treat. Although doctors can perform plastic surgery on some stretch marks, most cannot be treated in this way. A few doctors have applied dermabrasion to the scars. This procedure, however, has been soundly discredited by the rest of the medical profession. (For a further discussion of stretch marks and cosmetic surgery see Chapter XI, "Your Skin—Still Changing.") So what can you do to prevent scarring?

You can take preventive measures during your pregnancy—the earlier the better:

- Stay away from empty calories and watch your weight. Although each woman's resistance to stretch marks varies, the added five pounds can be the straw that breaks the elastic tissues' structure.

- Keep your skin well lubricated. It helps seal in moisture and prevents skin from drying out. Cocoa butter and moisturizing body creams applied two or three times daily are helpful in keeping skin supple. Pure bath oils help seal in the water absorbed from the bath.
- Don't massage your skin vigorously. This might damage your fragile tissues. Apply moisturizers gently.
- Exercise regularly. Exercise builds up abdominal muscles that help support the uterus. As we explain in "Your Pregnant Body—Staying Healthy and Fit," a good workout helps give you good skin tone by aiding blood circulation.
- One doctor we talked to recommended a pregnancy girdle that helps support the weight of the uterus and reduces stress on the skin of the abdomen. Ask your doctor about this.

DISCOLORATION OF THE SKIN. One pretty brunette friend was three months pregnant when she noticed something strange. While looking in the mirror she was surprised to see her face still had its deep tan, even though it was November and she hadn't seen the sun since August. As she further examined her body, she saw that her nipples and the areolas (the colored area around the nipple) were dark brown. A call to her obstetrician assured her that these skin changes were perfectly normal—especially in brunettes. Very fair-skinned and blonde women may find themselves with only slightly darker areolas. These skin color changes are thought to be caused by high levels of a hormone called human growth hormone (HGH) that triggers extra output of melanin, a protein that gives skin its color. Here are the most common skin discolorations:

*Mask of Pregnancy—Chloasma or Melasma.* The "mask of pregnancy," or chloasma, is the wintery tan our brunette friend noticed. It occurs more frequently in brunettes and black women, but no matter what your coloring you may discover you have brown or yellowish-brown patches on your cheeks, upper lip, forehead, or neck—all symptoms of this harmless hyperpigmentation. Sometimes the condition is so extensive the woman will actually have a raccoon "mask" look on her face: while the rest of the face is tan, the eyes and their orbits are spared because of their lack of melanin.

Black women sometimes develop white or "depigmented" patches on the face, neck, and upper back. These will usually disappear soon after delivery.

Chloasma can begin to show as early as the second or third month of pregnancy and usually fades within three months after delivery. Chloasma is often caused by birth control pills, too; if you do get it when you are not pregnant, your doctor should be notified.

Even if you don't already have it, the sun can bring on chloasma. One prominent dermatologist, Dr. Charles DeFeo, says the skin is often like undeveloped film waiting for the sun to develop it. If you do have chloasma during pregnancy, the sun will make hyperpigmentation much worse, deepening the discoloration five times faster than if you stay out of the sun. The sun may even make chloasma permanent—though most sun-deepened chloasma will fade if you avoid the sun completely.

Chloasma need not be a serious problem. For one thing, it's often really unnoticeable. One doctor we spoke to thought it looked "cute" on his patients and, to be truthful, in some cases it does. Even if you don't agree, you may rest assured that it usually goes away after delivery. Meanwhile remember the following:

- First of all, don't attempt to correct the situation with "peeling" methods, pigment reduction creams, bleaching creams, or any other methods at this point. These could do more harm than good. Wait until well after delivery, and see if the chloasma goes away.
- If you have bad chloasma and *have* to be in the sun, use a powerful sunblock. Zinc oxide is the best total sunblock sold over-the-counter. This white oily cover-up may look silly—but may be a life saver in certain situations.
- For most people, a good sunscreen containing para-aminobenzoic acid (PABA) is sufficient to block out the most harmful rays of the sun. Many suntan lotions are now coded to indicate their degree of protection. Choose a product marked 15 for greatest effectiveness. Remember to reapply your sunscreen peridocally, especially after swimming.
- Wear a wide-brimmed sun hat—even if you're just walking a few blocks to the office or the grocery store. The reflection from tall buildings can increase the sun's effect.

- If you find that walking around outside is causing the hyperpigmentation to become more noticeable, you can mix a sunscreen with your own moisturizer, or wear a foundation that contains a sunscreen. Many manufacturers include this product in their lines.
- Lips are particularly sensitive to the sun. Always wear lip gloss or lipstick when you go outside—lip glosses which contain a sunscreen agent are also available.

*Makeup Secrets for Covering Chloasma.* If your chloasma is slight but you'd like to hide it, follow these suggestions from Pablo Manzoni, New York makeup expert. (Pablo's makeover of pregnant model Lynne appears on pp. 38–43.)

a. Use a concealing cream or stick on the discolored areas—the kind you would use to hide dark circles under the eyes. Choose a color as close as possible to your own skin color, or no more than one shade darker. White or very light shades of concealing creams make the area look grayish or bluish. Use your fingertips or the stick to apply the cream to the area you wish to hide. Gently pat on a small amount at first. You can build up to more coverage by patting on additional amounts.

b. Next, apply a foundation over the concealing cream. Choose a foundation that covers well. A moisturizing foundation or an oil-based foundation will probably work best. A water-based foundation might mix with your perspiration and last only a few hours. Again, use a color which comes closest to your own skin shade.

If your chloasma is light, a foundation alone—without the concealing cream—might be all that is needed. Experiment with both techniques.

c. Apply your eye makeup, blusher, and lipstick as you normally would.

If your chloasma is very obvious and concealers and foundations don't do the trick, try COVERMARK by Lydia O'Leary. This opaque concealing foundation will help to mask any skin pigmentation. It was originally developed by Lydia O'Leary to hide her own facial birthmark. COVERMARK resists water and won't crack or cake. It also acts as a total sunblock.

Cosmeticians will give you a free consultation at Lydia O'Leary's salon in New York City. They'll help you choose shades and show you how to apply the makeup. If you can't visit, write for information and a color chart. Address: Lydia O'Leary, 575 Madison Avenue, New York, New York 10022.

*Linea Alba.* The "linea alba" or "white line" running from the navel to the pubic bone is barely distinguishable when you are not pregnant, but often becomes pigmented to a dark brown color during pregnancy. This is due to the human growth hormone (HGH) effect on melanin and occurs by the sixth month of pregnancy. It is then referred to as the "linea nigra" or black line. It sometimes extends beyond the navel up to the solar plexus. The line on the lower abdomen is often covered by hair ranging in color and texture from fine white to bushy dark. The linea nigra usually fades within a year after delivery. See Chapter XI, "Your Skin—Still Changing," for more information.

*Hyperpigmentation of Other Areas.* If you're a blonde or a redhead, your skin may not change color at all during your pregnancy. But ninety percent of us do see a very slight and generalized hyperpigmentation of all the skin as well as on the particular areas we've discussed above; and there are other areas which might darken during the course of your pregnancy:

> *The nipples and the surrounding areas, the areolas.* Doctors look for the darkening of this area as one of the first signs of pregnancy. The vulva (or external female genital organs) and the entire area extending from the urethra to the anus also darken. Darkened nipples, areolas, and vulva usually fade until they are close to—but never as light as—their original color within six months after delivery.
>
> *Freckles, moles, warts, brown spots, and recent scars.* All tend to darken, grow larger, or change in some other way during pregnancy.

Although moles and other spots frequently change due to hormonal levels, you should point out any changes to your obstetrician. Any bleeding from these moles or other skin marks should be reported immediately.

*The skin on the lower abdomen.* You may find it darkens and develops freckles.

SUN AND PREGNANCY. Beaches, sun, and water are a perfect setting for a pregnant woman. She looks a part of all nature about her. But how good is sun for the expectant mother?

The only *real* beneficial effects of the sun are a little vitamin D and the lift you get from looking and feeling good—temporarily. The adverse effects are broken capillaries, wrinkly, prematurely aged skin, or even skin cancer. Because of the increase in the steroids your pregnant body is producing, you will tan much more quickly than usual, so be careful. Wear a two-piece bathing suit if you like but don't get a dark tan on your tummy. Your abdomen will deflate when you have your baby and will look darker than the rest of your body, just the way a deflated balloon seems darker than one that's full of air.

If you have developed chloasma, stay out of the sun completely. The sun could cause the mask of pregnancy to become permanent—especially among brunettes and black women. (See "Chloasma," pp. 13–16.) Don't mix photosensitizers—antibiotics or perfume are two major examples—with the sun. They may make your skin more susceptible to the sun's ultraviolet rays, and you can get a terrible sunburn.

There are reasons other than proper skin care that should make you beware of overexposure. The more pregnant you are, the more dangerous long exposures to the sun can be. Since your body generates more heat of its own during pregnancy, sunstroke could occur more easily then. (And too much intense heat may be harmful to the baby.) If you're in doubt, less is best: have lunch inside and stay out of the midday sun.

For a tanned look without going in the sun, use one of the marvelous skin bronzers on the market. Bronzers are tinted gels. They give your face a tanned, healthy outdoors look without the risk of the damaging effects of the sun. Bronzers contain alcohol, so dry skin types should beware of using them every day.

ITCHING—THE MOST COMMON SKIN PROBLEM. Dermatologists see more itching, or "pruritis," than any other skin problem during pregnancy—usually during the latter four and a half months. Pruritis can take the form of a mild itch, or red bumps, or even severe eruptions complete with blisters; it is usually felt on the abdomen but it can spread to the breasts, buttocks, and all over. This itching problem peculiar to pregnancy is thought to be caused by a number of elements: among them dry skin stretched over your distended stomach; intense perspiration; even stress. If your case is particularly bothersome, consult your doctor; she may prescribe medication or medicated creams. If your itching is slight, simply slather on lots of moisturing cream. Fortunately, after delivery the condition almost always disappears.

There is another kind of common skin irritation you might have. Like two of the women we interviewed, you may have suddenly gained a lot of weight and begun to have a heavy person's problem—chafing thighs. If the skin on your thighs is red, use a light dusting of cornstarch to relieve the itch and irritation. Wear cotton slacks to keep your thighs separated. Wear light mesh pantyhose, but stay away from elastic pantyhose. They hold in moisture and could aggravate your problem. Leg exercises would be helpful in firming muscles and slimming down your legs.

UNSIGHTLY SPIDER VEINS—SPIDER ANGIOMAS OR SPIDER NEVAE. During pregnancy some women develop broken blood vessels that look like little red spiders at the side of their noses and on their cheeks, or, less commonly, on the shoulders, chest, and back. These are called spider veins—or spider angiomas or spider nevae—and they occur when a central arterial vessel dilates and little spidery legs grow out from the dilated center. You may also get a reddening of the palms—called Palma Erythema—along with these spider veins during pregnancy.

Two thirds of all pregnant women will get at least one spider angioma.

Among fair-haired, fair-skinned blue-eyed women, these veins are particularly noticeable. Some spiders may appear early in pregnancy but they do tend to increase until the time you give birth. Miraculously, they usually disappear or recede within six weeks after you've had your baby. (See Chapter XI, "Your Skin—Still Changing," for treatment if they persist.) As we said earlier, wait. Avoid facial massages, vigorous facial treatments such as "vacuuming," and electric current treatments. Don't treat them before you've given them a chance to go away. Be aware that the spiders crop up again—usually on the same site in subsequent pregnancies.

What can you do as an immediate remedy for spider veins? Cover and camouflage! Beauty expert Pablo Manzoni says, "It's easy to cover a vein. There are wonderful foundations today that you simply blend on—maybe with the help of a sponge. The finish is just so delicious and it looks as though you're wearing nothing."

Pablo also advises using an oil-based foundation rather than a water-based one. The oil-based foundation gives better coverage.

Use your foundation like a covering cream. Says Pablo, "Choose a shade very close to your own skin tone. Then simply cover the small areas affected by spiders."

SKIN TAGS. Among the odder occurrences pregnancy visits upon unsuspecting mothers-to-be are small growths called skin tags—flaps of skin that with some stretch of the imagination look like little tags. They can appear on breasts, areolas, the neck, and/or under the arms. They begin to appear after about four months. Skin tags usually remain after you have your baby. If you like, a dermatologist can remove them by cauterizing after delivery or, if they're on your breasts, after you've stopped nursing.

PREGNANCY AND ACNE. If you're at all troubled with acne, you'll be delighted to hear that pregnancy clears it up for many women. And fifty percent of those women whose acne disappeared during pregnancy will keep their clear skin after delivery. Pregnancy works for acne the way birth control pills do: both add estrogen to your system which slows the flow of sebum and counteracts the effects of androgen, the hormone that is thought to stimulate the oil glands. The added amounts of estrogen might give acne sufferers a boost over the last bit of acne they had.

On the other hand, there's also a possibility that the hormonal fluctuations of pregnancy—like those of adolescence—will make you develop acne, pimples, whiteheads, or blackheads for the first time in your life. If this happens to you during your first trimester, wait until the second trimester when your estrogen levels are high to see if your skin problems disappear. In most cases they do. If acne persists, it will usually get better after delivery—although some women have continuing problems.

If you develop skin problems ask your obstetrician to recommend a dermatologist. Acne can leave scars, so don't simply wait for it to go away. There are a number of topical substances (substances applied to the skin) that are considered safe for your baby and that should help clear up your blemishes. Your doctor might prescribe any of the following: vitamin A acid; antibiotic alcohol lotion; benzol peroxide; drying lotion; drying and peeling lotions; astringents and soaps.

Remember that no internal antibiotics should be administered while you are pregnant unless your condition is very severe and your obstetrician approves of it. Avoid tetracycline, the antibiotic usually prescribed for acne. It is known to give the growing fetus discolored teeth and bones. Erythromycin is considered a safe oral antibiotic but should be administered only if the condition is very severe.

Some dermatologists will also do acne surgery, expose the skin to quartz light, inject cortisone or steroid cysts, and take out blackheads.

For day-to-day skin care to minimize acne, follow the advice on pp. 21–24, as well as these general rules for acne sufferers (check with a dermatologist first):

- Get plenty of sleep; eat healthy foods; avoid stress; exercise and shower afterwards.
- Wash your hair four to six times a week with an acne shampoo to keep scalp and skin under your hair clean. If you wear bangs, wash them every day.

- Let inflamed pimples alone. Squeezing may infect them and your skin may be particularly sensitive during pregnancy.
- If you are normally allergic to any food, perfume, or other substances, be especially careful of them now. These irritants will only aggravate your acne.
- Don't treat acne with commercial preparations yourself. Acne caused by pregnancy is often different from other acne. See your doctor. She will give you medicated lotions and makeup if necessary.

TROUBLESOME OILY SKIN. One day Julia's husband gently suggested she stop using so much lotion on her face and forehead. "You're only twenty-four—you don't really need all that stuff on your face." Julia—who was three months pregnant—hadn't put a thing on her face. She realized she had oily skin for the first time in her life.

Oily skin—usually caused by hormonal imbalance or by the stress of changing your life-style to include a baby, or poor diet and rest habits—is not uncommon during pregnancy. You too may discover that you're suddenly troubled by large pores, whiteheads, blackheads, and occasional skin breakouts. Only parts of your skin may be affected. Perhaps the "T-zone" alone (forehead, nose, and chin) will be oily while the skin on your cheeks may even be dry. (See "Combination Skin," p. 25.) Test your skin for oiliness: wait two hours after you've washed your face and blot your face with a facial tissue. Use one tissue for each area of your face. Do you see residue oil on the tissue? If you do, that area is considered oily.

Here's a beauty program for oily skin:

*Cleansing.* Cleansing is extremely important for oily skin. Excessive oil on the surface of the skin leads to clogged pores. The skin then becomes infected more easily. If oil is not removed properly by cleansing, pores can become permanently enlarged. Cleanse your face (or other affected areas) two or three times a day. You might also visit an expert at a skin care salon or at a department store for advice on what products are best for your oily skin. Investing in a whole new skin care program can be expensive, so you should buy small amounts because your oily skin will probably clear up after delivery. And you don't have to dispose of all your old creams and makeup: if you had dry or normal skin before you were pregnant and now have oily skin, use your old moisturizer creams to lubricate your stomach, buttocks, legs, or elbows instead of your face. (One product you might not want to use is a hormone cream since the FDA has warned that hormones can be absorbed through the skin and can even reach the fetus—although many doctors doubt that creams are harmful if used moderately. If you decide not to use them, store them in your refrigerator until after the baby is born.)

Follow this cleansing routine:

1. Use an oily skin cleanser or a medicated soap to remove all makeup. Thoroughly cleanse your face. *Pat* dry with a clean towel.
2. With a cotton pad, apply a toner or astringent specially formulated for oily skin. Let the air dry your face.
3. Three times a week, use a grainy cleanser to help slough off dead skin cells. New York skin expert Mario Badescu has given us this natural, inexpensive recipe that you can make at home.

*Grainy Cleanser*

Mix together:
1½ tablespoons cornmeal
1 tablespoon milk

After washing your face with soap or cleanser, apply this mixture and gently rub into the skin with circular motions. Rinse with warm water.
In addition to cleansing, this will also help to tighten pores.

4. Use a commercial mask for oily skin two or three times a week. Buy a clay or a gel mask. Their deep cleansing and tightening qualities are especially good for oily skin. Mario Badescu gives two more recipes that you can easily make yourself. Alternate them during the week.

*Deep Pore Cleanser Mask*

Mix 1 teaspoon of dolomite (you can get this at a health food store) and enough fresh cucumber juice, tomato juice, or strawberry juice to make a paste.

Apply to face and leave on 10 to 15 minutes.
Wash off with tepid water.

*Pore Tightener Mask*

Mix together:
1 egg white
10 drops of lemon juice (the more lemon juice you add the tighter it will make your skin)
a little cornmeal (optional)

Apply and leave on for 5 minutes.
Wash off with warm water.

## *Beauty Tips for Oily Skin.*

- Don't overcleanse oily skin. Your skin may become dried out from using harsh skin cleansers and toners and the oil glands will start working overtime to replenish the supply. The result is skin oilier than you started with.
- Carry facial blotting papers or premoistened astringent pads to remove excess oil during the day.
- If you can, go without foundation—at least during the day. Foundation clogs pores. For the evening, use a water-based foundation or gel makeup rather than an oil-based or moisturizing foundation. The latter will only add more oil to your skin.
- Use a light moisturizer around the eyes. Even if the rest of your skin is oily, the eye area has very few oil glands and needs moisturizing.
- If your skin is very oily, your doctor may recommend one of the superficial peelers on the market. These mild chemical peelers remove the outer layers of skin so the new, fresh skin can appear.
- Consistency is the key. Follow your beauty routine faithfully. The brand of skin care products you use isn't as important as the regularity with which you use them.

*Product Checklist for Oily Skin*

- ☐ Oily skin cleanser or medicated soap
- ☐ Astringent or toner for oily skin
- ☐ Grainy cleanser for use two or three times a week
- ☐ Mask for oily skin
- ☐ Eye cream or moisturizer
- ☐ Medicated drying lotion for occasional outbreaks of acne
- ☐ Astringent pads or facial blotting papers for during the day

SUDDENLY DRY SKIN. Dermatologists tell us they see as much dry skin as oily skin during pregnancy, perhaps because the excess estrogen being produced by the placenta slows the flow of sebum or oil to the skin. Dry skin is characterized by flaking and scaling or blotchiness, usually on the cheeks.

Follow this beauty routine for dry skin during pregnancy:

*Cleansing.* The most important thing to remember about cleansing dry skin is to be gentle—with your beauty products and your hands. Avoid harsh deodorant soaps and astringents containing large amounts of alcohol. (You can tell if an astringent contains a lot of alcohol just by its smell.) Use your fingertips to wash your face and apply cleansers. Rubbing with a washcloth could cause your skin to become red and irritated. Here is a sample dry skin cleansing routine:

1. Wash face with a mild cleansing cream, cleansing lotion, or superfatted soap in the morning and at night.
2. After washing, apply a gentle toner formulated specially for dry skin.
3. Moisturize your face after cleansing and throughout the day whenever your face feels dry.
4. Use a rich eye cream before going to bed.

*Beauty Tips for Dry Skin.*

- Use an oil-based or moisturizing foundation.
- Use a clay mask or an enriching mask such as this one given to us by Mario Badescu:

*Mask for Dry Skin*

Combine:
1 egg yolk
½ teaspoon of olive oil or peanut oil
Blend until they are the consistency of mayonnaise.

Then add:
½ teaspoon of cornmeal

Apply this mixture to your face with a gentle circular motion. While the egg and oil are nourishing your skin, the cornmeal works to remove dead skin cells.

Allow the mask to remain on your face for 15 minutes and rinse off with tepid water. Follow with a moisturizer or night cream.

- Carry a lubricating eye stick in your purse to use throughout the day.
- Invest in a special night cream to use on your face and neck. Pablo Manzoni recommends alternating two night creams so that your skin never gets used to just one.

*Product Checklist for Dry or Normal Skin*

☐ Cleansing cream, cleansing lotion, or superfatted soap
☐ Mild toning lotion
☐ Moisturizer
☐ Eye cream and lubricating eye stick
☐ Mask for dry skin
☐ Night creams

COMBINATION SKIN. During pregnancy many women often find themselves with a "combination skin" problem—skin that is a combination of oily, dry, and normal. The most common combination skin type is that in which your T-zone remains normal or oily while your cheeks become dry. For this problem, simply use the suggestions under "Dry Skin" for the affected cheek areas. Use the suggestions under "Oily Skin" for other areas that have become oily. This double program may seem troublesome but treating a dry area as an oily area or vice-versa could have damaging effects on your skin.

DEEP CLEANSING FOR ALL SKIN TYPES. Pregnant or not, the basis for all beautiful, healthy skin is *clean* skin. Regular daily cleansing usually doesn't "deep clean" adequately. Deep down dirt should be removed every once in a while. Now that you're pregnant, why not pamper yourself and have your skin cleaned at a professional skin care salon? It's a relaxing and delicious treat—especially in the latter months of pregnancy when you need a lift. Ask questions so you can apply their techniques at home.

Most salons follow the same skin care routine:

- The best part comes first—your trained cosmetician gently massages your face and neck with a cleansing cream. You'll find this treatment relaxes you and relieves facial tension.
- Next your face is steamed with a gentle mist or herbal sauna.
- Then two different types of cleansing masks are applied.
- Next your cosmetician will clean out your clogged pores and blackheads.
- A moisturizer finishes off the facial. You're beautiful and your skin is dazzlingly clean.

*How to Give Yourself a Facial Sauna at Home:* This is fun and inexpensive, but it can be drying. If your skin is dry already, limit the duration of your saunas; and in any case do not use them more than once a week.

- Pull your hair off your face. You can set hair in large pin curls and the steam will help it curl.
- Cleanse your face with soap or cleansing cream. Remove excess cream.
- Heat a large pot of water on the stove.
- When the water begins to boil, take the pot off the burner. Place it on the kitchen counter. *Never risk getting burned by putting your face over the pot while it is still on the fire.*

- Place a towel over your head to make a tent and lean over the pot, staying about 18 inches away from the water.
- Let the steam cleanse your face for five to ten minutes—no longer. You will have to come up for air occasionally.
  (The steam is good for the mucous membranes in your nose and throat, too!)
- Dry skin beware! Steam your face only two or three minutes.
- Follow sauna with a mask and then a moisturizer.

FACIAL HAIR AND HIRSUTISM. One phenomenon of pregnancy that might affect the skin on your whole body as well as on your face is hirsutism or excess hair. It's rare, to be sure: our friend Jill's obstetrician had heard complaints of excess facial hair only a few times before. Upon examination of Jill's cheeks and upper lip the doctor did see some fine blond hairs—nothing very noticeable. But Jill insisted she was growing more hair all over her body and had new peach fuzz on her face since she was pregnant. What could she do about it?

There is a chance that Jill was growing new excess hair. Although excess hair—or hirsutism—is not very common during pregnancy, sometimes the hormonal upheaval or perhaps the increased body temperature of pregnancy does cause it. Hair on the upper lip may grow fuller and darker. Hair on the arms or the legs, hair around the nipples and areolas, and the fine hair on the cheeks may increase.

One dermatologist we spoke to said hirsutism does occur during pregnancy but since women are more aware of their bodies at this time they might simply be noticing their facial hair for the first time. "Pregnancy is like summertime," says Dr. Hillard Pearlstein, assistant clinical professor of dermatology at Mount Sinai School of Medicine. "Suddenly you're in a bathing suit and you begin noticing all the little moles and bumps and hairs you never thought you had."

Our advice for Jill is to wait. For any excess facial hair that persists after delivery, talk to a dermatologist and see our advice in Chapter VIII, "Your Body Postpartum."

FEELING HOT. "I was carrying Peter in one of the coldest winters on record," said one of our friends, "but I felt hot and perspiry all the time!"

Most of us feel warm during pregnancy—for a very good reason. Our temperature rises at least one degree due to elevated progesterone levels during pregnancy. The sweatiness results from an increase in the activity of eccrine—or sweat—glands, which are helping to rid both you and your baby of waste products.

Beneficial though this process is, it can be uncomfortable at times. So what can you do about excessive perspiration? Try these:

1. Take a long extravagant bath at least once a day if the doctor approves. Do this at night so you can get rid of all the waste material accumulated during the course of the day. (See "Bath," pp. 30–33.)
2. Wear loose clothing that allows your skin to breathe, and stick to natural fibers. Cottons are wonderful while you are pregnant; synthetic fabrics often block air passage.
3. The only place you really need a deodorant is under the arms. Use a roll-on or cream deodorant. Stay away from aerosol deodorants containing possibly harmful chemicals especially while you are pregnant.
4. Air is great for the skin! When you have a few moments alone in the privacy of your home, take off all your clothes, lie down, and let the air cool your body. Air is also a terrific stimulant and toner for the skin. Make sure your room is warm and there are no drafts to cause chilling.

THE CAESAREAN SECTION. The last mark your pregnancy might make on your skin is the scar left by surgery for the delivery of your baby by Caesarean section. (See Chapter VII, "Your Hospital Stay.") An incision is made in the abdominal and uterine wall to remove the baby in some cases of breech presentation, placenta previa (in which the placenta is placed abnormally near the cervix), disproportion between baby and mother, and other medical complications. More than one in ten of us winds up having her baby by Caesarean, and that percentage is on the rise.

Nancy is one of these women; she traveled two hundred miles to New York City to have her Caesarean deliveries. Why? "The doctors in my area

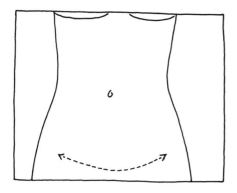

The "bikini" cut.

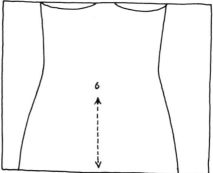

The vertical cut.

don't do 'bikini cuts,' " she explained. "Why should I have to wear a one-piece bathing suit for the rest of my life to hide my Caesarean scar when a bikini scar hardly shows even when I'm naked?"

The most important cosmetic consideration of a Caesarean delivery is the surgical cut. There are two methods of Caesarean surgery. The bikini or Pfannensteil cut that Nancy wanted is a horizontal cut starting at the pubic hairline, dipping down and following the line across the lower belly where a bikini could easily cover it. The vertical cut extends from just below the navel to the pubic bone and leaves a very noticeable scar when it heals.

Many women prefer the bikini cut for obvious reasons, and some doctors feel it heals faster than the vertical cut, is less likely to produce a hernia, and less likely to rupture in subsequent pregnancies. Through our interviews with doctors we found that the only reason to have a vertical cut is *speed.* If the baby is in distress and has to be removed immediately the familiar vertical cut is often used. Even then, an obstetrician trained to do a bikini cut can often perform it just as fast as the vertical incision. With fetal monitors and other advances in obstetrics, there is more time than formerly to perform a bikini Caesarean. Our advice is: *shop around for an obstetrician who is trained to do a bikini cut.* If your obstetrician thinks your desire to show less scar is frivolous, that may tell you something about your obstetrician. It is amazing how resistant the medical profession is to change. Your desire to look good is as important as other considerations if the alternatives are arbitrary.

If you're having a second or subsequent Caesarean, you might also consider the technique Dr. Gideon Panter uses on his patients. For subsequent Caesareans, Dr. Panter removes the old scar tissue from the first Caesarean. He then takes out more tissue and, in effect, takes a tuck in the abdomen. The tummy is flatter and less flabby after delivery.

"I always talk to my patients before their Caesareans," says Dr. Panter, "and ask if they want a little less in this area. I haven't been turned down yet. I even remove some of the stretch marks by doing this—not all, of course. I think all women should ask their doctors about this 'plastic surgery' along with repeat Caesareans."

So do we.


## A TIME FOR BEAUTY

Now that you're pregnant, the ritual of beauty takes on special significance. You are the one who is in control now: you can establish and have fun with a routine of regular beauty care, or you can let the discomforts and troublesome side of pregnancy get you down.

Follow the lead of those around you who give you special attention at this time and *pamper yourself!* Although you may be a modern, active woman working at a full-time job, you are a lady-in-waiting and deserve this extra pampering. Give yourself this luxury—the world of skin care and hair salons await you. And the special time for beauty care at home should also be yours. Here are some wonderful ideas on how to indulge your body and spirit.

THE BATH—YOUR AT-HOME BEAUTY SPA. Showering is a fine way to keep clean and refreshed. But there's something about taking a long, lovely bath—while you're pregnant—that renews and reenergizes your body, mind, and soul.

Madolyn, a beautiful twenty-seven-year-old mother of one, had uncomfortable abdominal cramps when she was seven months pregnant. "Morning and nighttime baths saved me. My body felt like it was floating and the cramps disappeared."

Water supports the uterus and gives you buoyancy. The warmth of the bath increases circulation and relaxes the muscles, which tend to cramp during pregnancy. Your muscles have increased tone to cope with carrying extra weight and therefore cramp more easily. Taking a bath also gives you private time—time and space in which you feel free of demands. Children, husbands, aunts—all know that when Mommy is taking a bath you leave her alone.

The first pregnancy gift you might give yourself is a rubber mat or rubber decals for the bottom of your tub. They will prevent slipping—especially in your latter months when your body becomes surprisingly unwieldy. When you're getting in or out, support yourself by leaning against the wall and grasping the safety bar. During the last month or two, you may feel safer taking a bath when your husband or another adult is around to help you in and out of the bathtub.

Make your bath cozily warm—not really hot. Overheating your body may lead to birth defects in your baby. Hot water also stimulates your heart unnecessarily and encourages broken capillaries on your skin. To make matters worse, it also dries out your skin unmercifully. Soaking too long—even in a less-than-hot tub—dehydrates the skin and removes the natural skin oils, so watch your time. And use a pure, mild soap (avoid deodorant soaps because they are drying) and remember that too much soaping can also dry skin.

Here are some ways to make your bath especially wonderful while you're pregnant.

- Buy a pretty bath pillow covered in floral vinyl—or use an eyelet pillow filled with herbs to rest your head while you luxuriate in your tub. Or sew up your own pillow and fill with potpourri. The scent of the pillow mixed with the steam of your bath will fill the room with a heavenly fragrance. These little indulgences will make you feel like a queen—or at least a lady-in-waiting.

- You may be tempted to sprinkle in fragrant bath oils or bubble baths to make your bath even more luxurious—but don't. They might irritate your delicate perineal and vaginal areas, which are newly sensitized by being pregnant. Avoid all bath products containing perfumes and bubbling agents. Dr. Panter advises, "Remember that a pregnant woman has a swollen vulva and much more sensitive vagina. The tissue is redder because there are more blood vessels there. They can absorb more and are more likely to get an allergic reaction." Instead, stir up invigorating beauty baths by adding one of the following: a handful of sea salt; or a cup of oatmeal; or a cupful of oil of almonds. A milk bath is one of our favorites (perhaps because of its motherly overtones!). Pour in a pint or more. You'll love the silky way it makes your skin feel. Or use pure baby oil or nonscented bath oil in the tub to seal in moisture as you emerge from your bath.
- Pay careful attention to your elbows, knees, backs of arms, or any other areas that tend to develop rough, scaly skin. It may be harder for you to notice these areas—especially close to your due date when your body is so bulky you can't even see your feet. Your husband and others can still see them, so stock up on polyester or loofah sponges sold in drugstores. Buy sponges with long handles that permit easy access to legs, arms, knees, and back. These sponges remove the dead skin cells on the outer layer and allow the new clear and smoother skin to show through.
- A warm bath with a handful of Epsom salt thrown in is the perfect place to relax and soothe tired, achy leg and foot muscles. (See "Pretty Feet," pp. 36–37, for more ideas.)
- At the beginning, the bath or shower is a convenient place to shave your legs. However, by the last trimester, you may be too big to carry this off successfully. Try sitting on a toilet with your legs propped up on a stool. If you find you're nicking your legs too much, use shaving cream or baby lotion. Use a new sharp razor blade. If you are right-handed and have trouble reaching your left leg to shave, use an electric razor held by your left hand. The electric razor will prevent cuts when held by your inexperienced left hand. The best solution of all is to have your legs waxed professionally. It will make you feel indulged, and besides the obvious benefits of not having to shave

your own legs, you'll be amazed at how smooth and sleek they feel.

- Follow your bath or shower with an application of a moisturizing baby lotion—especially if you don't care for bath oil. This locks in moisture and makes your body even softer. Slather it on while your skin is still damp. Use moisturizers all over, but especially on your growing tummy and breasts. For hot days, keep a bottle of moisturizing lotion in the refrigerator and smooth it on your body right after your bath—it's cooling and sensual.

- Wrap yourself up in a soft terrycloth robe. (You may have to borrow your husband's by this point!) It will act as a sauna to allow the good oils and creams to be absorbed into the skin. Give yourself five more minutes on your bed, in front of the TV, or in a rocker to savor the last glow from the bath's warmth.

Most doctors consider showers safe even after you've gone into labor. However, obstetricians differ in their opinions about when to discontinue baths. Ask your doctor for her advice. Many will now allow a bath up to the time you start labor or your membranes rupture—unless you have bleeding or certain vaginal infections. More conservative doctors ask their patients to stop taking baths six weeks or more before their due date. They feel that if there is a slight possibility of infection when the vagina is exposed to bath water, you shouldn't chance it.

*Checklist for the Bath*

- ☐ Rubber bath mat or rubber decals
- ☐ Pure, mild bath soap
- ☐ Bath pillow
- ☐ Unscented bath oil or natural additives such as sea salt or milk
- ☐ A polyester or loofah sponge
- ☐ Callus reducer
- ☐ Pumice stone
- ☐ Moisturizing body lotion

PREGNANCY SCENTS. When you're looking so great during pregnancy, you want everything about you to be special—including the aura about you.

Perfume gives the finishing touch to your makeup and beauty routine.

Our only advice is to avoid using perfume on breasts and, as we mentioned earlier, in the genital area since the tissues are too sensitive. You may find your favorite perfume smells a little different on you. An expert on scents reports that the hormones secreted during pregnancy could affect the secretion of materials on the surface of the skin. Your skin could be more acidic or less acidic than it usually is. You may be eating a different diet, the protein makeup of your skin might be changing. All these factors might change the way a fragrance smells on you. The way things smell to your nose also changes—especially during the first trimester—so this too may account for your new perception of your old cologne.

This is a perfect time to experiment with new scents. If you've been using a lemony scent, try a woodsy or spicy one. Try something new, something exotic, some fragrance you never dared wear before.

### "SMILE—YOU'RE PREGNANT!"

A beautiful smile that shows healthy, gleaming white teeth is especially lovely on a pregnant woman. Fear not that pregnancy will threaten the health and look of your teeth since the old wives' tale, "a tooth for every baby" (you will lose one tooth for every baby you carry) is simply not true. The baby does not decalcify the mother's teeth—you will be providing his calcium needs with a calcium-rich diet. (See "Calcium," p. 77.)

Here are some tips on caring for your teeth during pregnancy:

- Brush your teeth two or three times a day as you normally would. Some women feel too nauseated even to look at toothpaste in the morning. If so, try brushing with baking soda or salt and warm water, or even plain water to remove bacteria and food from your teeth.
- Use dental floss to remove any food that might be lodged between the teeth.

- Visit your dentist early in your pregnancy to clear up any dental problems you may have. Inform your dentist that you are pregnant. Only local anesthesia should be used. X rays should not be done unless your dental condition is severe. Use a lead apron if X rays are necessary.
- Many women find that their gums bleed during pregnancy. This is a very common condition known as "pregnancy gingivitis" or inflammation of the gums. The hormonal flux of pregnancy can cause the membranes of the gums to puff up and bleed. This inflammation can last for months and usually clears up completely after delivery. In the meantime, see your dentist and use a soft toothbrush to remove food particles from the affected area. A salt water rinse is also recommended for gingivitis.

2113261

## GREAT NAILS—ANOTHER BONUS OF PREGNANCY

"See, my nails are turning all my friends green with envy," said eight-month-pregnant Evy to the pregnant women at her prepared-childbirth class. "Mine are pretty terrific too," said Caroline, waving her beautifully manicured nails in Evy's direction. "And for the first time in my life."

A chorus of "Mine too" followed—each one of the women in the class had long and pretty nails, the product of seven or eight months of nail- and hair-boosting hormones of pregnancy. Nails are made up of keratin, like hair. In fact, they *are* another type of hair. (If you're past your ninth week of pregnancy, your baby has begun growing his nails too.) If you find you've got lovely nails for the first time in your life, or if they've just improved and you want to show them off, get a professional manicure or do them yourself. Polish up. As one of the delightful beauty assets of pregnancy, pretty manicured nails should be flaunted.

Edema may be one problem of pregnancy which puts a damper on the look of fingernails and toenails. Your hands and feet may be anywhere from a little to very swollen from mild edema. If this is your problem, don't hide!

Proper nail care will beautify the total look of your hands and feet. Follow these tips: (1) Let your fingernails grow slightly longer than you would normally. The longer nail slims the look of your swollen fingers. (2) File fingernails into a smooth oval shape. Don't file them straight across—this will only make your fingers look chubby. Keep toenails filed neatly. Try to get an oval shape to even the contrast between toes and nails.

Avoid bright and very dark nail polishes. Make your fingers look longer and your feet less swollen by using lighter shades, such as dusty rose, light plum, or the more natural earth tones.

## PRETTY FEET

What a workout your feet endure during pregnancy—especially toward the end! Your feet have to bear all the extra weight of pregnancy and are often swollen with edema. Many women find they have to go to the next size shoe (see Chapter V, "Fashion During Pregnancy"). As feet spread, and pressure is exerted on them from added weight, calluses develop and fallen arches are not uncommon.

How can you care for and beautify your hard-working feet? Here are some suggestions:

TOENAILS. Since your toenails, as well as your fingernails, are growing faster, you will probably need a pedicure more often than usual. It is easy to overlook the toenails since they are not as accessible and not easily viewed with your large stomach. Remembering that they grow faster and need cutting more often will help prevent problems with ingrown or injured toenails.

Toward the end of pregnancy you may have to get a professional pedicure since your big stomach presents a logistical problem in doing your toenails. You can also have your husband or a friend help you. Use a clear nail polish for toes since colored nail polish requires too much upkeep.

CALLUSES. The bath is probably the best place to care for calluses and corns. Toward the end of your bath use a callus reducer for the calluses on the soles of your feet. Use one with a rough mesh surface to remove dead skin softened by the warm bath. For more sensitive areas of the feet use a pumice stone.

FOR TIRED FEET. Methods for relaxing tired feet are not only medically sensible but are also downright sensual! Here are some suggestions:

- Elevate tired feet whenever possible. Do foot circles (see below) to increase circulation to the feet. Do these as often as possible throughout the day, particularly if you are troubled with poor circulation in your legs and feet.
- Alternate hot and cold foot baths. Spend about one minute in each one, ending with a cold bath. Do this three times a day if necessary.
- Powder feet librally before putting on shoes.
- Have your husband or a friend give you a *foot massage*. It is one of the most luxurious things you can have done for you. Thousands of nerve endings are located in the sole of the foot so when you massage the feet you stimulate all the rest of the body as well.

   Prop your feet up on a pillow and have your helper use a little oil or body cream on your feet. Your helper can follow these instructions:

1. First massage the sole of the foot by making a fist with your right hand while holding the foot with your left. Make small hard circles with your knuckles, going over the entire sole.
2. Then hold the foot in both hands with your thumbs on the sole. Work both thumbs in small circles over the entire sole. Switch your thumbs to the top of the foot and work them in the same way.
3. Next the toes. Hold the foot with your left hand and the base of the big toe with your right hand. Gently pull the big toe with your thumb and forefinger, twisting slightly from side to side until your fingers slide off the toe. Repeat for each toe.

## THE BIG SPLURGE!

By your ninth month, you'll have experienced any skin change you're going to experience at all. Most likely you'll look very beautiful—as well as *very* pregnant. You're probably feeling a little anxious and restless and definitely ready to burst. Now is the time to make the big splurge. Make an appointment at a beauty salon or for someone to come into the privacy of your home a week or two before your due date. Concentrate on *you* instead of what's coming. Get the works! It's fun to have your hair styled, to get a facial, a manicure, and a pedicure. (Stay away from colored nail polish as nurses must check the skin under nails for any possible lack of proper oxygen when you are in the hospital.) If you'd like a massage, be sure to go to someone who is experienced in working with pregnant women. You can also get a beauty makeover at the salon. Do it all—you deserve it.

PREGNANCY BEAUTY MAKEOVER BY PABLO MANZONI, MAKEUP EXPERT. Here's pretty Lynne, eight months pregnant, all set for her makeover by Pablo Manzoni. "I'm feeling very good, but also very big and a little tired," says Lynne. "My eyes and lips have become a little puffy in the last few months and my face is fuller than it's ever been before. This makeover came just at the right time. I can use a little lift right now."

Pablo tackles Lynne's problems and gives easy makeup solutions. If you have similar problems, adapt his ideas for your own makeup. You have more time to experiment while you're pregnant than after, so now is the time to try new looks you see in fashion and beauty magazines.

Some women tend to pile on a lot of makeup while they're pregnant. But why hide or compete with your beautiful rosy glow? Try not to use a heavy hand when you do apply your makeup. You're already somewhat larger and heavy makeup can make you look clownish. Stick to natural shades and tones—you'll look better for it. Go somewhat dramatic at night if you like, using more color on your lips and cheeks and eyes.

Make sure your skin is very clean when you begin your own makeup (see our cleansing programs for all types of skin on pp. 21–26). Pablo sug-

# · PREGNANCY BEAUTY MAKEOVER ·

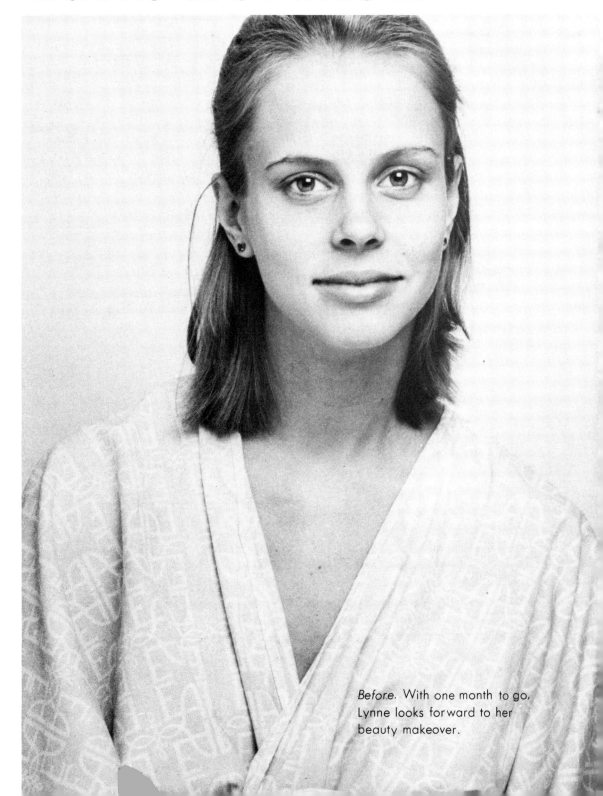

*Before.* With one month to go, Lynne looks forward to her beauty makeover.

gests that you keep eyebrows shapely by tweezing under the eyebrow and never allowing hair growth between the eyes.

Women who have allergies may find themselves more allergic to cosmetics during pregnancy—but some women are less allergic during pregnancy, and others stay the same. Even if you are not allergic you may find that the odors of some lipsticks, foundations, etc. make you feel queasy—especially in the first trimester. Discontinue using these products. You might want to try one of the cosmetic lines that does not contain perfume.

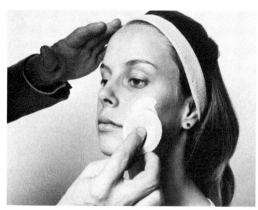

*Step 1—applying moisturizer.* First Pablo applies moisturizer with a sponge. "I always work with sponges," says Pablo. "They're softer and kinder than one's hands." If your skin has become oily during pregnancy you may not need a moisturizer at all.

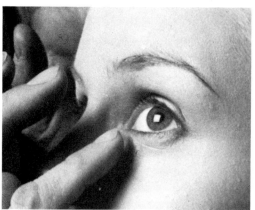

*Step 2—applying foundation.* Next Pablo applies a soft beige foundation to Lynne's face. The sponge enables him to carefully blend the foundation (especially around the jaw line) so that no demarcation can be seen.

Pablo daubs a small amount of concealing cream on his pinky and, while Lynne looks up, gently pats underneath her eye, starting at the inner corner, patting outward until blended.

Pablo suggests using a concealing cream and a little extra foundation around the nose or cheeks if the pregnant woman has spider angiomas. You can also use extra foundation around the nose to cover any open pores. Pablo advises, "Use foundation to cover what you don't like—such as uneven skin, a rosy glow that's too ruddy, or other imperfections. However, if you have good skin, don't bother with foundation."

If you find you have dark circles under your eyes, you can usually correct them at this stage. Dark circles result from too little sleep or poor diet. In late pregnancy, one always seems to be fatigued. The color drains from the face and the circles look even darker in comparison. Pablo covers Lynne's circles with a concealing cream. He says, "Concealing cream should never be used all over the eye area because we don't have dark circles on the *outer* part of the eyes."

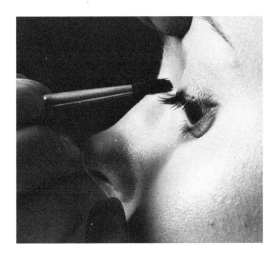

*Step 3—Lynne's eyes.* Pablo has chosen a plum-colored cream eyeshadow for Lynne. He smooths it over the entire lid, leaving it darker at the outer corner.

Next Pablo takes an eyeliner and draws a very fine line close to Lynne's eyelashes. Then with a clean brush (see photo) he smudges and lightens the line. He repeats this process twice more. "You don't see a line," says Pablo. "But you see the presence of liner. This helps one's eyes look larger without having shown that you've used liner."

Then comes plenty of mascara on the top of the lashes and underneath too. Reapply another coat or two to make lashes look their thickest.

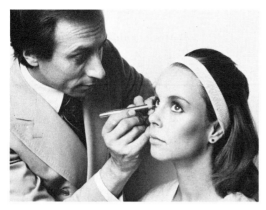

Pablo takes his famous "blue pencil" and lines the inner edge of Lynne's bottom lid. "It's practically my signature," says Pablo. "I love the way it makes the whites of eyes look whiter—it really brightens the whole eye."

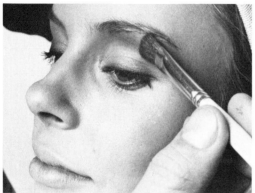

To correct the puffiness around Lynne's eyes, Pablo uses a brown eyeshadow on the bone line above her eye. Pablo says, "Brown eyeshadow is a miracle. I seldom do makeup without it. It corrects any problems and flatters as well." If your eyes are very puffy, extend a rich brown eyeshadow such as deep walnut over the entire eyelid, lightening as you approach the brow.

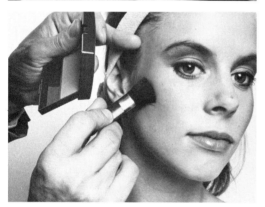

Step 4—Blusher. For Lynne's slightly fuller face Pablo applies the blusher on the highest part of the cheekbone and continues up to the temple. Avoid blushing the fleshy part of the cheek right under the eye. This makes your eyes look puffier. A cream rouge in combination with a powder blusher makes the color last longer.

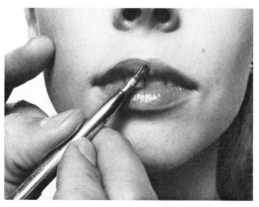

Step 5—Lips. Lynne had full lips to begin with, but—as often happens—pregnancy made them even fuller. Pablo prefers using a clear or a light-colored gloss to deemphasize the fullness. Here he softens Lynne's lips with a clear gloss and then brushes on a plum gloss. Pablo recommends piles of rich gloss to brighten your face all during pregnancy and prevent chapped lips.

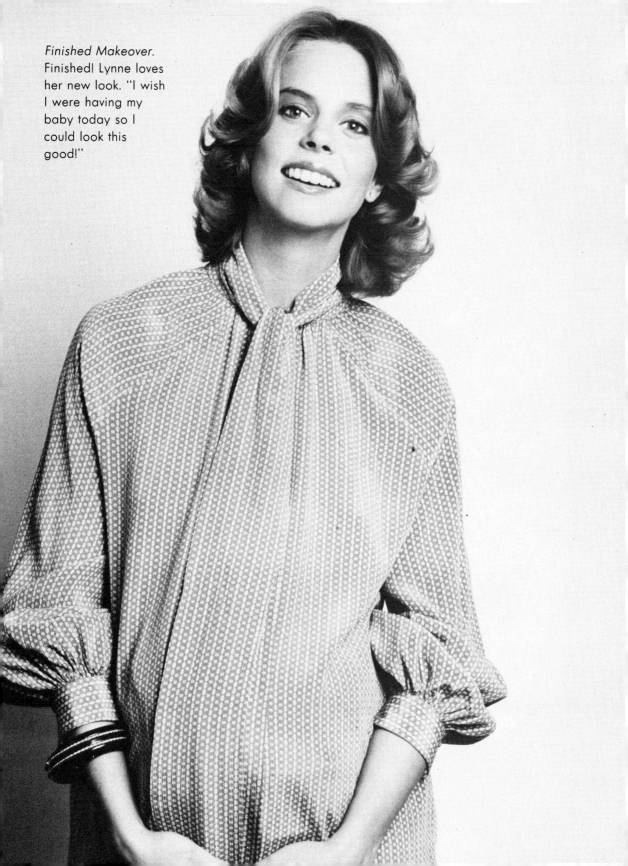

*Finished Makeover.*
Finished! Lynne loves
her new look. "I wish
I were having my
baby today so I
could look this
good!"

## WHAT ELSE CAN I DO FOR MY SKIN?

The old adage, "beauty comes from within" is not far off—especially when a woman is pregnant. But that inner glow of happiness can go just so far unless the other important elements are there too: proper diet, regular exercise, sufficient rest, and freedom from stress.

DIET. All the makeup and beauty care products in the world can't begin to match the wondrous effects you can work on your skin all by yourself. And your skin care program doesn't have to cost a cent. A later chapter discusses how important a good diet is to your health and that of your growing baby, but the food you eat has an effect on your skin, which needs to be nourished with proper nutrients and vitamins. Stick to your own rules— you know your skin best. However, be on the alert for new food sensitivities during pregnancy. Hormonal changes may cause your skin to react differently to certain foods.

All the good that added estrogen does for your skin during pregnancy is undone by smoking and drinking. Both slow down blood circulation and cause your skin to retain waste materials. They keep your skin from really glowing and looking its prettiest. They actually cause premature aging of the skin. For your skin's sake and your baby's sake, try to cut down or quit both at this time.

EXERCISE. If you've ever seen someone who has just completed a good workout, you know what exercise can do for the look of skin. That wonderful glow and great color come from increased circulation and can't be matched by any shade of blusher. Since pregnancy increases total body fluids as much as thirty percent because of water retention and larger blood volume, exercise is essential for good circulation. Exercise also tires you out and makes you sleep better.

SLEEP. Sleep is one of the best beauty tonics. Now that your body is working overtime to produce your child, it is even more important. You know how terrible your skin can look when you're run down. Now is a special

time to take care. Steal as much sleep as you can, starting in the early
months of pregnancy. If you're working, get to bed earlier each evening.
Put your feet up in the office whenever you can.

AVOID STRESS. Skin experts tell us that they often see the effect of stress on
the skin. Skin problems flare up during periods of anxiety and worrisome
situations. We know that pregnancy can be a stressful time for all women.
So for your skin's sake and your own mental health try to minimize your
stress by talking about your fears and anxieties, setting aside a quiet time
during the day to pamper yourself, and not forgetting that sex is one of the
oldest and best tension relievers.

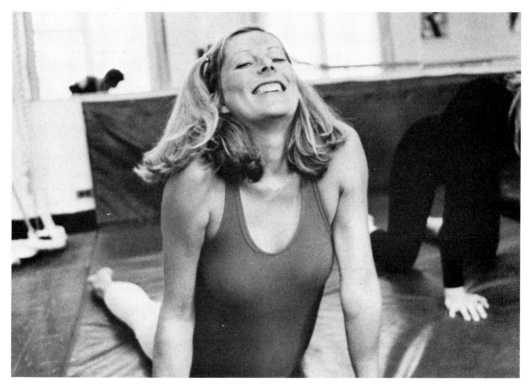

An added bonus of exercise is healthy, radiant skin.

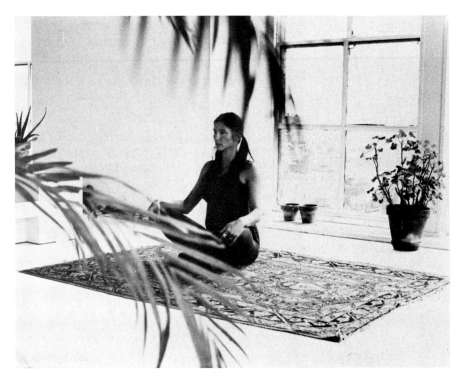

Many pregnant women meditate to relieve stress and relax their bodies.

## LASTING BEAUTY

Great skin doesn't just happen—you have to make it happen. Each time we spoke to a pregnant woman whose skin looked lovely, she invariably told us that aside from the natural glow pregnancy bestowed, she cared for it in a special way. The extra care you give your skin at this time shows the world you feel good about yourself and your pregnancy.

Now is the perfect time to establish a skin care routine that will last and last—especially through those first few hectic months after the baby is born. The time you spend now will save time later and make you feel and look terrific these nine pregnant months.

# CHAPTER · II ·
# Hair — How It Can Be Your Best Beauty Asset During Pregnancy

"WHAT'S GOING TO HAPPEN to the texture of my hair during pregnancy? Will it be straighter, curlier, thicker, softer, more oily? Will it take a permanent or color differently?"

"I'm so tired of the way I look. I need a change—should I get my hair cut?"

"My face is so full. I've gained weight and have a little edema. What are some nice hairstyles to offset my fuller face?"

"I've heard your hair falls out after you have a baby. Is there anything I can do to prevent this?"

"I'm hot all the time and my long hair constantly bothers me. I don't want to cut it. What should I do?"

If one of those questions sounds like you, you'll find the answers here. Pregnancy is a time when your hair *can* look the best ever—but sometimes it seems like so much trouble. Washing, drying, or curling your hair when you feel tired or clumsy—especially in your last trimester—can be drudgery instead of a delightful beauty ritual. But it doesn't have to be that way. We've found ways to minimize the problems and let the natural beauty of your hair take over—because we know that if your hair doesn't look good you don't *feel* good.

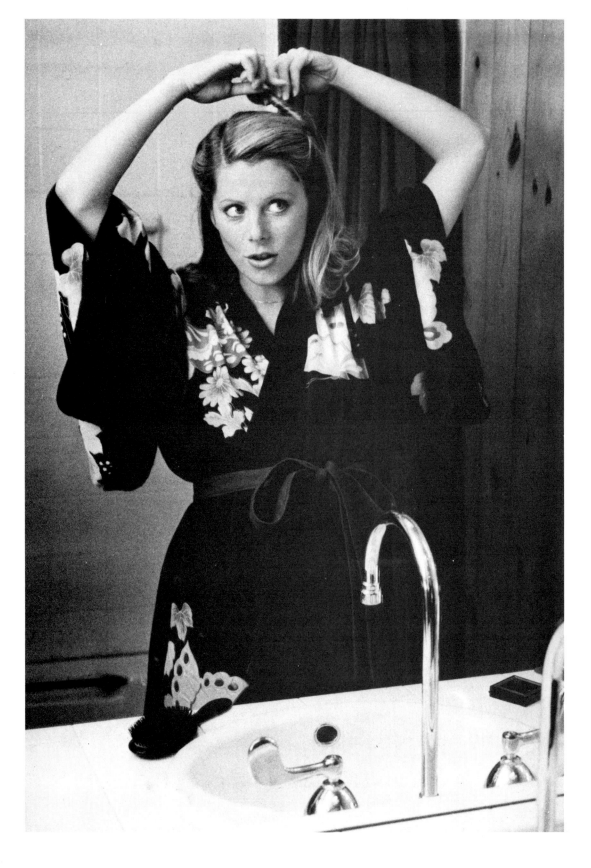

## YOUR HAIR'S "GOLDEN AGE"

Almost all of the women we have talked to reported that the look of their hair improved during their pregnancy. This discovery is borne out by a 1973 study ("Changes in Hair and Skin Condition During Pregnancy," published in *The British Journal of Clinical Practice*—see the Bibliography at the back of the book) that showed that, of a group of 131 pregnant women, "between one third and half the group noted changes in the gloss, feel, appearance, and body of their hair, the majority of them recognizing an improvement."

How does pregnancy make hair look so much better, better than your late teens when your hair was supposedly its thickest and healthiest? The answer has partly to do with hair growth patterns. As you probably know, the hair on your body is dead. It is the follicle located in the scalp at the base of the hair that is alive. Hair is made of keratin, a ninety-percent fibrous protein substance. At any given time—outside of pregnancy—ninety percent of your hair is in the "growing" or "anagen" phase. The hair follicles are actively producing keratin, or hair. This growing phase lasts from three to six or seven years for each hair. Then the "resting" or "telogen" phase begins. Ten percent of your hair is in this stage at one time. It lasts three to six months. During this stage hair growth stops. Its attachment to the base of the follicle is weakened, and out comes the hair. Of the approximately 100,000 hairs on your head, about 100 are lost each day. After the hair falls out, the follicle then grows new hair, once again beginning the "anagen" phase.

This process is the *normal* hair growth cycle. During pregnancy, however, hormones affect changes in the normal growth pattern so that beginning between the thirteenth and fourteenth weeks of pregnancy, usually *more* than ninety percent of the hair follicles stay in the growing phase and *less* than ten percent of the hair continues in the resting phase. During pregnancy you've just got more hair! Furthermore, studies have shown that there is an increase in the percentage of thick hairs grown during pregnancy.

This wonderful news doesn't, alas, apply to everyone. There are a mi-

*Opposite page:* Twist it, braid it, crimp it, just play with it. Your hair should be at its best during pregnancy.

nority of women (some of whom took oral contraceptives just before their pregnancy) who report duller, less lustrous hair, more split ends, or more greasiness.

Whether your hair is giving you problems or whether it looks better than it ever has, now is the time to develop a good hair care program.

"You know, now that my hair looks so great," said five-month-pregnant Jean, "I'm giving it more attention. It's like slender people—they're always dieting and exercising. I'm going to make my good thing even better." Hairdressers agree. The better care you give your hair now, the better shape your hair will be in during the crucial postpartum time. In the two to six months after delivery most of us lose a small to a significant amount of hair (see pp. 294–300). You can't do anything to stop this, but you can

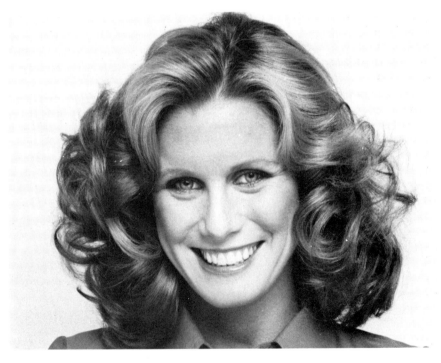

Pregnancy hormones bolster hair body, making it thicker and more lustrous—perhaps the prettiest it's been since your teens.

make sure that the hair that remains is in tip-top shape. And this takes planning right now, during pregnancy.

Besides getting thicker and stronger, what else can happen to your hair in these nine months of change? The texture of the hair may alter slightly. Although dermatologists and hairdressers have not indicated that pregnant women's hair becomes curlier or straighter, some women we spoke to noticed these changes. A few women with naturally curly hair reported that their hair became less frizzy during pregnancy. The study cited earlier reported that some women complained that during pregnancy their hair did not take a set as well as it normally did. And others have said that their hair reacts differently to permanents. Try a strand test if you have any doubts. But remember that in general hair texture seems to change more drastically *after* birth. (See Chapter XII, "Hair—Quick Solutions to New-Mother Problems.")

The biggest change you might experience is a sudden oiliness or dryness, caused by the new hormone levels your body is coping with. When you've had normal hair all your life, a change to oily or dry hair or the development of a troubled condition during pregnancy can be perplexing and irritating. It's an annoyance you simply don't need at this busy time of your life. If it happens to you, try one of the following programs designed for women who are suddenly experiencing dry or oily hair. You might also talk to your hairdresser about commercial products to aid your condition.

WHEN HAIR TURNS DRY OR BRITTLE DURING PREGNANCY. Hair experts, such as Philip Kingsley, a British trichologist (one schooled in the art of hair analysis), see more dry than oily hair during pregnancy. In fact, they see enough dry hair on pregnant women to offer helpful advice. Dry hair is brittle, develops split ends easily, damages and breaks off easily. Although it can still look thick, it will be dull, even lifeless. What to do about it?

*The Cut.* Get yourself a terrific haircut or trim. A good cut is extremely important for all types of hair—but even more so for long dry hair. Long hair is old hair and there is greater potential for dry, split ends. A trim every six or eight weeks will give shape and body to dry hair and eliminate split,

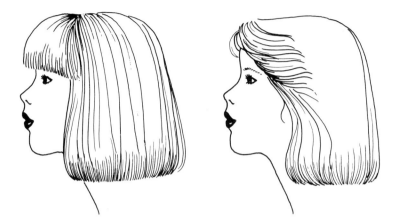

This medium-length cut is perfect for dry hair and offers great versatility at the same time.

cracked ends. Try to get a cut that will allow you to dry your hair naturally, without the use of blow dryers or curlers.

*Shampoo.* Choose a very mild shampoo such as baby shampoo or one formulated especially for dry hair. Wash hair every three or four days. Lather only once and be sure to rinse out all the shampoo. (A good rule of thumb is, rinse hair until you feel it is thoroughly clean and then rinse again for one more minute.)

Take special care when combing wet hair. Wet hair is very elastic and will stretch and break if not handled gently. Be sure to use a wide-toothed comb on wet hair to remove tangles.

*Hot Oil Treatment.* Dry hair responds very well to a hot oil treatment. Warm a small amount of light vegetable oil—or one of the many convenient ready-to-use hot oil treatments on the market—and work into hair and scalp. Wrap hair in a warm, wet towel and cover with a plastic bag. Leave it on for an hour or more. Remove bag and shampoo. Lather hair twice to wash out all the oil.

*Conditioning.* Give yourself a serious conditioning treatment once a month with a commercial conditioner—not a conditioning rinse but a cream or pack that is left on the hair wrapped in a wet, hot towel for ten to twenty minutes. In addition follow each and every shampoo with an instant conditioner that is left on the hair for one to three minutes.

*Blow-Drying.* After a shampoo, allow hair to air dry completely whenever possible. If you don't have the time, allow it to dry partially. Then use a blow dryer to finish it off. Choose a dryer with no more than 800 to 1,000 watts to avoid damaging the hair. In order to avoid further dryness, stay away from styles that require blow-drying every day. Try one of the conditioner/hair moisturizer products formulated to be used with blow dryers and electric rollers.

*Electric Rollers.* Save electric rollers and curling irons for special occasions. Don't use them every day. Always use end papers with electric rollers.

*Brushing.* Use a natural bristle brush. Brush only when your hair needs it. Keep strokes to a minimum number. If you have a curly hairstyle, try easing the curls into place with your fingers for a more natural look instead of brushing.

*Massage.* Some hair care specialists we spoke to recommended gently "finger massaging" the scalp in order to increase circulation and oil flow. The benefits of massage are debatable. But if you like the way it makes you feel, it can't hurt!

*Chemical Treatments.* Hair coloring, bleaching, permanents, and straightening are all processes that work on the molecular structure of the hair. They weaken the hair, often leaving it dry and brittle. Avoid them whenever possible.

*Hair Spray.* Hair spray tends to dry out hair. Use as little as possible or avoid completely.

WHEN HAIR TURNS OILY DURING PREGNANCY. One common change in hair during pregnancy is the development of oily hair. This is a possible result of the sebaceous glands in the scalp being overstimulated by high levels of certain hormones in the bloodstream during pregnancy. What are the indications that you have oily hair? Your hair looks as though it needs a shampoo one to two days after you have shampooed. It may also look a little matted within a short time after you shampoo. It lacks body and bounce. Here's what to do.

*The Cut.* The best cut for oily hair is one that is simple to care for. Let your hair be itself—if it's curly, wear it curly. A good cut should give sharp definition to hair and allow it to fall into place with a few flicks of your comb.

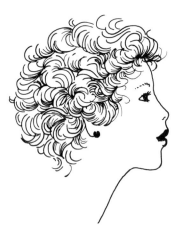

If your hair is naturally curly and oily, this cut is a no-fuss style for easy care during pregnancy.

*Shampoo.* The best way to deal with oily hair is to shampoo frequently. You may have to wash it every other day or even every day. If you're afraid this may be hard on your hair, remember that models wash theirs almost every day—and they look terrific!

Use a mild shampoo for frequent washings. If you find you need a stronger shampoo to get your hair really clean, try one made especially for oily hair. Don't fall into the trap of using a harsh shampoo. This could strip so much oil from your scalp that your sebaceous glands will work overtime to replenish its supply and you will end up with an even oilier scalp and perhaps dry, split ends. If you find that a shampoo is effective one week and doesn't seem to be doing the job the next, switch to another shampoo. Alternate two or even three different shampoos.

*Conditioning.* If your hair is healthy though oily, you won't need to use a conditioner. Don't let any advertisement lead you to believe that you do! If you're not conditioning, use a shampoo that contains protein for extra body.

You *will* need a conditioner when the ends of your hair are dry or split. Apply the conditioner to the ends of your hair only. Don't work it into the rest of your hair and scalp. Comb through and rinse well.

If you don't need a conditioner, but find it difficult to comb your hair out after a shampoo, put a very small amount of conditioner in a large glass of water. Pour mixture through hair and rinse out immediately. This small amount of conditioner will make your hair easier to comb, but won't leave excess oil on your hair.

*Vinegar Rinse.* You might want to try this age-old beauty treatment after you shampoo. Mix a ½ oz. of apple cider vinegar in a large glass of water and rinse through hair. Wash out with warm water. This is excellent for removing any residue soap or oil, and it actually seems to unsnarl tangles as well. It leaves hair bouncy and shiny.

*Blow-Drying.* If your hair is in good condition, it can be blown dry every day. After washing your hair, comb to remove tangles. Let your hair "air dry" for 10 to 15 minutes, then blow dry, moving the dryer all over your head. Never hold the dryer on one piece of hair for more than a few seconds.

*Electric Rollers.* Electric rollers and curling irons can be used as you need them when you have oily hair. Always use end papers with the rollers.

*Brushing.* The best brush for blow-dry styling your hair is the kind with a hard rubber base and firm plastic bristles. This type holds up well under lots of heat.

For general use, the natural bristle brush is a good choice. It is very gentle on hair. Look for a brush with hard bristles if your hair is thick, and soft bristles if your hair is fine. Forget about the 100 strokes a day rule. Excessive combing and brushing will stimulate the oil glands unnecessarily.

*Massage.* Massage is definitely out if you have oily hair. It will only activate glands to produce more oil.

*Chemical Treatments.* Oily-haired people do have an advantage when it comes to hair coloring, permanents, and straightening. Their hair is usually stronger and better able to withstand the drying effects of these processes. In some cases, hair coloring can actually improve the look of oily hair. Whenever hair has been processed, however, it must be treated carefully and conditioned after every shampoo.

*Stress.* Keep in mind that stress and anxiety can possibly lead to increased oil production, as we mentioned in the "Skin" chapter. Stress can possibly aggravate an oily hair condition.

## STYLING

As your body and even your face become fuller during your pregnancy, you may find that you want a change from your tried-and-true hairstyle—for reasons of comfort if not for aesthetics. But what kind of change? And how much of one? We've put together some of the most-asked questions on the subject below: is one of them yours?

Q. I have long hair and I'm six months pregnant. What can I do with it when I feel so hot nearly all the time?

A. Long hair can act like a blanket in warm weather or during pregnancy when the body temperature is slightly elevated. The best solution is: Get your hair off your neck by pulling it up into a topknot, ponytail, braids, or roll. Liz (photo) has found a beautiful, classic look for her long hair during her pregnancy. She starts by loosely gathering her hair into a pony tail with a covered rubber band (less breakage!) at the back of the top of her head. She then twists the hair into a soft bun and secures with straight bobbypins. Liz pulls out a few loose curls to add softness around the face and neck.

Long hair pulled back into a ponytail with pretty ribbons always looks neat and fresh. Or try braiding long hair in one long braid intertwined with gingham, grosgrain ribbon, or a narrow piece of leather.

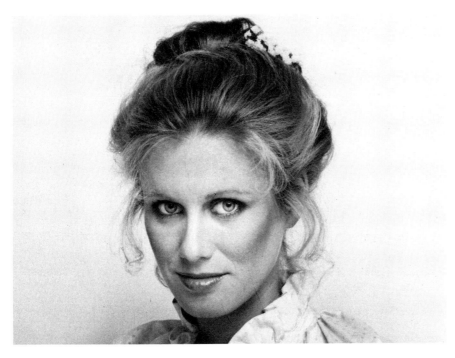

Feeling warm or overheated is one of the most common complaints of pregnancy. Here's one of the best hair solutions for this problem—an all-year-round classic and lovely look.

Rolling the hair (see sketch) is a great look for day or evening. If you find it too difficult to do yourself, have your hairdresser roll your hair for you. It's less expensive to go to the salon with freshly washed and dried hair. Your hairdresser will style it for you in a roll, braids, or whatever you like.

If you are pregnant in the warm months and you find the humidity and the perspiration on your scalp leaves your hair damp and limp, try washing your hair more often. Follow our hair care program for dry or oily hair depending on your hair type.

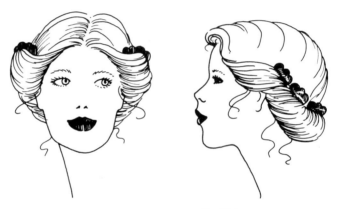

Combs add a pretty touch to "rolled" hair.

Q. I'm five months pregnant and have long hair. My problem? My hair has to be blown-dry and styled each time I shampoo. I get so tired standing on my feet holding the blow dryer for twenty minutes at a time. My stomach also gets in the way when I have to bend over. What can I do?

A. This is a tiring process for any woman and especially so for a pregnant one. Here are some tips that can help:

- If your hair is very long you might consider having it trimmed to shoulder length. It will still look long, but won't take as much time to blow dry.

- Invest in a dryer that comes with a holder and can stand by itself on a table. You can then sit down to dry your hair. Move the dryer around or move your chair around to dry each section of your hair. You can watch TV, do needlepoint, or manicure your nails while your hair is drying. Do your styling at the very end when your hair is still damp.
- Try letting your hair dry naturally. It's better for the health of your hair. Style your hair while it is slightly damp or set in electric rollers.
- Set your hair in regular rollers and sit under a home hood-style dryer. These portable hood dryers may be a good investment for you now and after the baby is born as well.
- For a new look, try setting your hair in small braids while it is fairly wet. Let it dry for a few hours. Your hair will come out with a pretty "crinkled" look.
- During the week, look for specials at your local beauty salon for wash and blow rates. Let someone else do the work for you!

Q. I'm so tired of doing my hair in rollers or blowing it dry. I want to try a permanent. I had one years ago and loved it, but can I have one while I'm pregnant? Will my hair take the wave?

A. A friend of ours went for her semiannual permanent when she was three months pregnant and all she got were bends and kinks—to her horrified surprise. When she went back to her hairdresser a few months later, obviously pregnant, she complained about her previous permanent. "If you had told me then that you were pregnant," her hairdresser said, "I never would have recommended a permanent."

Most of the hairdressers we spoke to had observed that permanents often do not "take" on pregnant women the way they do on nonpregnant women. In fact, French hairdresser Pierre Ouaknine of Pierre Michel Coiffures in New York was astonished to see American hairdressers giving pregnant women permanents at all. Pierre said, "In Europe, numerous hairdressers prefer not to give pregnant women permanents because they feel they just don't take well." The hairdressers and dermatologists were at a loss to explain why exactly this happens but, once again, hormones seem to be the culprits.

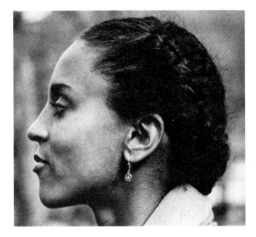

Alva has a terrific hair trick for busy working mothers-to-be. She shampoos and gives her hair an application of coconut oil. (Many black women have naturally dry hair or dry hair due to straightening or overprocessing—coconut oil restores life and shine.) Alva then puts her slightly damp hair up in braids. She goes off to exercise class or to do errands.

By the time she begins her modeling work, Alva's hair is dry. When she combs it out, she's got a dramatic hairstyle for an elegant daytime or evening look.

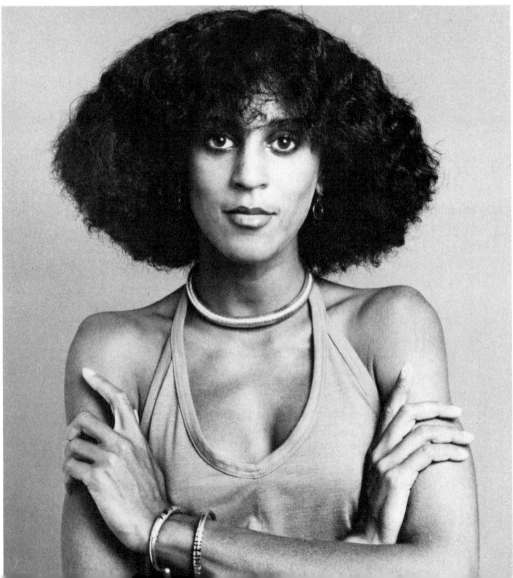

Not every pregnant woman with whom we spoke had unusual results with perms. One hair expert said it was in fact an excuse hairdressers used for giving poor permanents. Whatever the reason, be aware that a permanent might fail during your pregnancy. You might want to wait till after you deliver.

Q.  My face seems so fat from weight gain and edema. Which hairstyles are best for me now?

A.  Try following these dos and don'ts:

*Don't*

- Pull hair back into a tight ponytail. This shows off a full face.
- Pull hair straight back on the sides with combs or clips—save this style for after you have your baby.
- Cut hair very short.
- Wear hair long and straight. This style makes the face look even rounder.
- Wear bangs that come straight down on your forehead. This shortens your face and makes the lower half look fuller.

*Do*

- Create *some* fullness and uplift in your hair by using electric rollers or a blow dryer.
- Choose a soft, simple style such as the medium length shown in illustration. (Severe or graphic cuts or hairstyles emphasize a full face.)
- Create some interest around the forehead with soft bangs swept back.
- If you do choose a shortish style, make sure it has fullness and an upsweep at the sides.

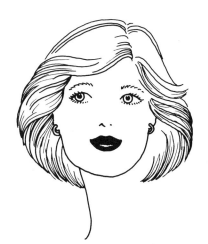

This softly layered cut has the clean, uncluttered look that is flattering for the slightly fuller face.

## TO CUT OR NOT TO CUT?

The most dramatic change you can make in your hairstyle is to cut it, a course which seems increasingly attractive if you suffer from the heat, are tired of rollers and blow dryers, and are desperate for a carefree new look. But before you decide to part with your glorious locks of hair during pregnancy or to adopt a new, shorter style for once the baby comes, consider these questions:

| YES | NO | |
|---|---|---|
| ☐ | ☐ | 1. Have you ever had short hair before? |
| ☐ | ☐ | 2. Did you think it looked well on you? |
| ☐ | ☐ | 3. Have you been spared the "full face" look mentioned earlier in this chapter? |
| ☐ | ☐ | 4. Do you think short hair will go well with your new pregnant figure? |
| ☐ | ☐ | 5. Will you be content with one basic style rather than having the flexibility that long hair gives you? |
| ☐ | ☐ | 6. Will you have the time and energy to shampoo and blow dry every day if your short hair requires it? |
| ☐ | ☐ | 7. Does your husband ever admire women with short hair? |

How many nos do you have? More than two? If so, reconsider cutting your hair much shorter than it already is. Many women cut for the wrong reasons. They are depressed and want to change or they feel it might be easier to take care of. Consciously or unconsciously women may feel that a short haircut is more fitting for a new mother. It's as though they are prepared to leave their old status as a sexy woman behind on the salon floor to become a sensible mother. (After all, doesn't your mother have short hair?) One friend's husband was furious when his pregnant wife came home with a short haircut after years of wearing it at a medium length. "Nora," he fumed, "every woman I know who's gotten pregnant has had her hair cut short! I thought you would be different!"

Short hair can be a happy change while you are pregnant and often a perfect solution for a new mother's tight schedule in many cases. But first look at the questions you answered no to:

1. If you've never had short hair, don't cut it now. Pregnancy is not the time for such a dramatic change.
2. If you wore your hair short two years ago and really didn't like it then, there's no reason to think you're going to like it more now. Don't let a hairdresser talk you into a short style just because he thinks it's the "look."
3. Short hair makes the face appear fuller. If your face is already slightly bloated from edema, a short cut could emphasize its fullness. If your face hasn't gained weight and your complexion is good, a short style definitely gives your face a "lift." In many cases you'll look younger without a lot of hair pulling your face down.
4. Remember that your pregnant figure will probably be quite large toward the end. There should be a nice balance to your silhouette between your face, hair, and body. Short hair can give you a pinhead look if the rest of your frame is large.
5. Most short styles offer little opportunity for variations. As great as a short style can look, it will look the same every day.
6. Many short styles have to be washed and blown dry every day to hold their shape.
7. Husbands are not always the best critics when it comes to their wives' hair and often resist *any* change in their wife's appearance. But, also consider the fact that your husband is seeing a lot of changes in you during these nine months. If you've always worn long hair, a short cut might be too much for both you and him. Wait till after you have the baby to make a big change in your appearance.

## BLEACHES, HAIR DYES, HAIR SPRAYS, AND OTHER POSSIBLE HAZARDS

There may be some risk in dyeing or coloring your hair. In the past, National Cancer Institute tests showed that certain ingredients used in some hair colorings were a possible cancer hazard. (These substances can be absorbed through the scalp into the bloodstream during the coloring process. The risk becomes compounded when you are pregnant, since a child may also be affected: harmful ingredients in the bloodstream can cross over the placenta to reach the fetus.) Hair color companies have removed these ingredients from their products and are confident that their products are safe, although the Environmental Defense Fund contends that substitutes for the suspected carcinogens and other ingredients in hair dyes have not been adequately tested and continue to pose a possible health risk, especially for pregnant women and their unborn babies.

The obstetricians we interviewed were divided in their opinions about whether to continue or discontinue using a hair dye during pregnancy. Many felt that the amount of dye used was not significant enough to affect the mother or baby. Other doctors felt that if there was any chance of harm, especially to the baby, a woman should avoid hair dyes during pregnancy.

Don't forget that hair coloring includes dyes, semipermanent dyes, and rinses. Hair color should "take" the same when you're pregnant as when you are not.

ALTERNATIVES TO HAIR DYES. Popular highlighting techniques such as streaking, tortoiseshelling, or sunbursting are good alternatives for two reasons—they need to be done only every five or six months, and they cover less hair. Another method of highlighting is streaking just the tips of the hair to give a "sunkissed" effect. This technique is recommended because the coloring ingredients do not touch the scalp at all.

If you want to avoid all chemical treatments while pregnant consider some of the *natural* products used to color hair.

*Henna.* Henna is a natural hair coloring that comes from the roots and leaves of a flowering shrub from the Middle East. This pure coloring agent has been used by women for centuries not only to color hair, but to condition it as well. Henna gives a natural color, brings out your own highlights, and adds body. Henna is not usually successful in covering gray.

*Camomile.* Camomile tea in strong concentrations can be applied to lighter shades and graying hair to give it blond highlights. Here's a lovely recipe that New York models have picked up from their Swedish sisters: Buy some loose camomile flowers. Brew them in a teapot with some water. Let the mixture cool and then apply the flowers and tea to your hair. Leave it on for 15 minutes. Rinse and style!

*Lemon juice.* Lemon juice may also give blond highlights. After shampooing and before going into the sun, take the juice from three freshly squeezed lemons and apply it to your wet hair. Let it dry in the sun or, if there's none available, under a strong light source such as a sunlamp or a 100-watt bulb.

SPECIAL TREATMENT FOR COLORED HAIR. Remember that bleached or colored hair needs special treatment. Hennaed hair can also become dry and brittle when treatments are too frequent. Condition and care for hennaed hair as you would for colored hair.

Use shampoos designed especially for color-treated hair and condition after every shampoo. At least once a month, use a deep penetrating conditioner. If you are going to use a hair dryer be sure it is on a low temperature setting.

ARE HAIR SPRAYS SAFE? Up to the time of this writing, no tests have been done on the effect of aerosol hair sprays on the development of the fetus. However, there have been other tests conducted which indicate that hair sprays shouldn't be used during pregnancy—and perhaps never. These tests show that inhaling hair spray—it's almost impossible not to—slows the rate at which the lungs clear themselves of mucus. The resins contained in most hair sprays remain in the lungs as well as the liver and spleen. Some propellants presently used in aerosol hair sprays are suspected to be carcinogenic, and the fetus is more susceptible to the effect of carcinogens.

So, why not give up hair spray? Hairstyles today are natural and "unset." They usually don't need hair spray. Hair spray does cause hair to get dirtier faster. If you can't live without hair spray, be sure to use it in a well-ventilated room.

## FOR HEALTHIER HAIR

Hair is an excellent barometer for the overall state of your health. Poor diet, lack of sleep, and severe stress eventually result in lackluster, limp hair and, in extreme cases, hair loss. A proper health program is the answer for healthy, shiny hair.

DIET. Hair is a handy tool for doctors who want to analyze your nutritional status. Believe it or not, insufficient nutrition, especially protein deprivation, shows up on your hair before it shows up in any other area—even blood. This is because the body "considers" hair one of the least important areas to direct protein to. Calories are also directed to other places than hair. This is especially true during pregnancy since the body has new needs— those of nourishing a growing fetus. The hair and skin will be the first to show the effects of a poor diet during pregnancy or at any other time.

Iron-deficiency anemia sometimes shows up in hair during pregnancy. Your obstetrician will be monitoring your hemoglobin count to see if you have enough iron. If you don't, anemia can cause many medical problems, as well as limp or graying hair.

As everyone knows, pregnancy is not the time to diet. A well-balanced nutritional program with vitamins and iron for pregnancy are all that are needed for shiny, healthy hair. Avoid such supposed cure-all formulas for dry or oily hair as brewer's yeast and vitamin B. Avoid megavitamin therapy—especially vitamin A. This can make your hair fall out, your skin dry, and cause all kinds of problems, including fetal defects. Discuss all vitamin intake with your doctor during pregnancy.

REST. Fatigue can also show up on your hair. Not getting enough rest inhibits the proper function of hair follicles. Limp and often dry hair can result. Proper sleep and rest are important to all phases of your pregnancy—even your hair.

STRESS. Whether stress affects hair growth or loss during pregnancy or at any other time is a controversial issue. Many doctors feel there is no hard

# · A WHOLE NEW LOOK ·

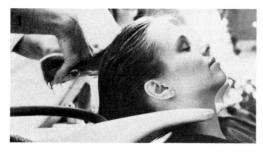

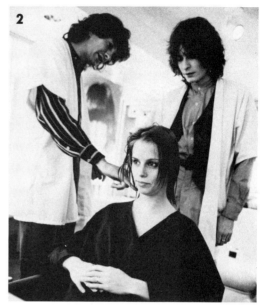

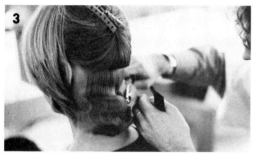

**1**   In the last month of pregnancy, Lynne relaxes and fully enjoys the luxury of having her hair shampooed, finger-massaged, and carefully combed. Having your hair done is wonderfully relaxing for all expectant mothers—a luxury worth saving for—especially late in pregnancy.

**2**   Didier and Patrick of Jean Louis David, New York City and Paris, consult with Lynne about her needs. Didier says, "I personally think when a woman is pregnant she is the most beautiful. Lynne is a perfect example."

**3**   Lynne did not want a permanent, so Patrick crimps Lynne's hair with a curling iron. As you see in the picture, the hair is first sectioned. The crimping is done on the bottom layer of the hair first and is continued upward. The two sides are done next and the top is done last.

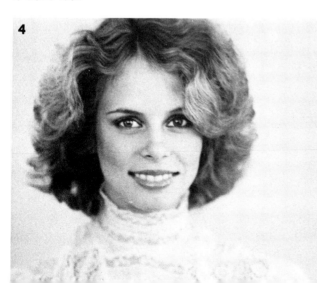

**4**   The effect is soft and romantic. The style is one that fits Lynne's mood at this time of her life— serene and feminine. She chooses an antique blouse full enough to wear over a long brown crushed-velvet maternity skirt, to complete the romantic image.

evidence that stress affects the condition of your hair. On the other hand, British trichologist Philip Kingsley says, "I'm a great believer that stress is one of the prime factors in hair and scalp problems." We do know that someone who is under a great deal of tension can develop "alopecia areata," a condition in which hair falls out in patches and in rare cases does not grow back. Try to relax and enjoy this special time.

If you take good care of your hair while you're pregnant, chances are you'll feel and look better all around. At no other time in your life will your hair be so glorious—so wear it proudly. And *baby* your hair. It may indeed be your best beauty asset at this time.

# CHAPTER · III ·
# Diet and Nutrition
# During Pregnancy

"WHEN I FOUND OUT I was two months pregnant," said Barbara, a new mother, "the first thing I thought was, 'What have I been eating and drinking these last months? Oh no—I took two aspirins last week. I hope it didn't affect the baby.' Being pregnant forced me to reevaluate everything I ate and drank."

What we put into, and have put into, our bodies should be and usually is the most immediate concern of newly pregnant women. Good nutrition and avoiding chemicals and drugs is the foundation for a healthy and beautiful pregnancy as well as a healthy and beautiful baby. Healthy, in this case, *means* beautiful.

## WHY EVERY PREGNANT WOMAN NEEDS TO EAT WELL

In fact, you may have to put aside other traditional standards of beauty; for while someone who gains only ten pounds during her pregnancy may be more aesthetically pleasing than someone who gains thirty, the former could be putting her baby and herself in real danger. Women who gain very little during pregnancy tend to have low-birth-weight babies, weighing

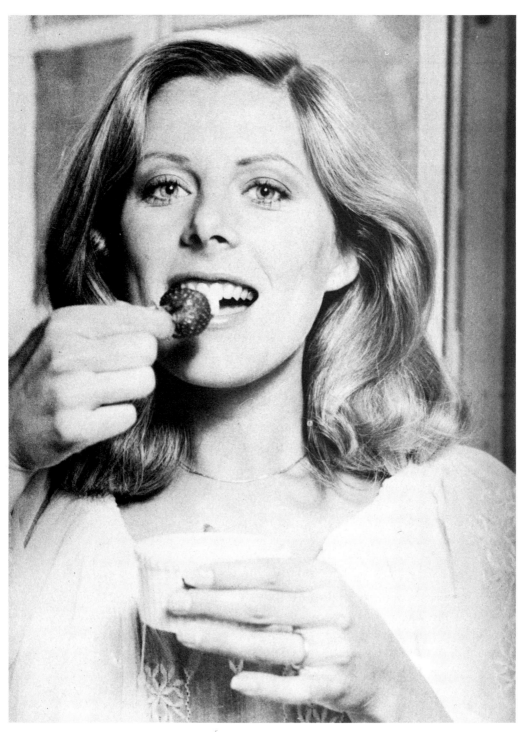

Joanne's indulgences are healthy. She dips a ripe strawberry into honey-sweetened yogurt for a nutritious snack.

less than five and a half pounds at birth. These babies are more susceptible to physical and mental disorders—some not appearing until age five or six. You may have a friend who restricted her weight gain carefully, put on only twelve pounds, and had a perfectly normal baby, but you may not be so lucky.

We were astounded at the number of women we interviewed who actually dieted during pregnancy. Women who were well educated and well informed were restricting their calories to 1,000 a day. And their doctors tolerated and even encouraged these eating habits! There's been so much research indicating that the restriction of caloric intake results in low-birth-weight babies, toxemia, and even the mysterious killer disease of pregnancy, eclampsia (see p. 73), that permitting these diets is now immoral and inexcusable.

On the other hand, gaining *too* much weight is not good for you or your baby either. It taxes your cardiovascular system and it's murder trying to shake it after the baby is born. Of all the pregnant women with whom we spoke, the ones most pleased with themselves and their figures were the women who were very disciplined about their eating habits. Many felt they were "in training" during these nine months and after. They ate very well, never skimping on the right foods and at the same time avoiding second helpings and the wrong kinds of food. If it takes the average woman 2,000 calories a day to maintain her weight, she needs to add only 300 more each day for pregnancy (more if she exercises regularly and vigorously), according to the National Academy of Sciences' "Recommended Daily Allowances."

The message in this chapter is to eat a *varied* and *well-balanced diet.* Include *more protein* and *more calories* (a minimum of 2,300 for the average pregnant woman) and other necessary nutrients while avoiding chemical additives and the empty calories of candy, other sweets, and junk food. While no sensible nutritionist will advocate indiscriminately gaining lots of weight, don't ignore or try to suppress your body's signals for more food. At no time in your life is nutrition more important than during pregnancy. Why not rethink your food habits now and start a new lifelong program of good eating habits? Your body, beauty, energy, and baby will all benefit from your careful attention.

This chapter explains why you need to eat well during pregnancy, how much of which foods you need every day, why certain foods, vitamins, and minerals are necessary to your baby's development, and what happens if you do not get proper nourishment. The usage of salt, a controversial topic, is also discussed. Weight gain is another complicated subject. How much should you gain? What if you were heavy or underweight when you got pregnant? We've given ideas for preparing your food and cutting down calories. We've also included sample menus and recipes. And if you have problems such as nausea and heartburn, see our dietary remedies.

This chapter also gives advice on what to avoid during pregnancy. Certain medications and food additives can have serious effects on your baby. We've listed these substances and their effects. There's also information on alcohol and smoking. Some of the most toxic teratogens (substances causing birth defects) surround you in your house. See our "Household Danger" list for information. Read this chapter carefully because good nutrition is important to your health—and especially your baby's.

THE FETUS IS NOT A PARASITE. "It doesn't matter that I don't eat enough of the right foods one day or the next, because a baby always takes what it needs from the mother's body," was the phrase used by many mothers we interviewed. But the concept that the fetus will extract whatever nutrients he needs such as calcium from your teeth and bones, protein from your muscles and other tissues, etc., may be just a myth that has been passed down from mother to daughter and friend to friend. It reassures the dieting pregnant woman that her baby will be fine no matter what she does or doesn't eat.

"The fetus is not a parasite," says Dr. Pedro Rosso of the Institute of Human Nutrition of Columbia University. "As a matter of fact, when a woman does not have adequate nutritional status during pregnancy, the baby is always proportionately more affected than the mother."

Dr. Tom Brewer, a physician who has researched malnutrition (and a pregnant woman on a 1,000-calories-a-day diet for more than just a few days at a time *is* malnourished) and its effect on pregnant women and their babies, further underscores this point in his and Gail Sforza Brewer's *What Every Pregnant Woman Should Know* (see Bibliography). "If the mother fails to take in all the essential nutrients in large enough proportions to sustain the increased demand of pregnancy, her baby will not magically receive what it needs for optimal growth. The baby does not have top priority for nutrients. In fact, there are numerous reliable studies which show the opposites."

YOU ARE EATING FOR TWO. The old adage, "I'm eating for two," was briefly discredited by doctors after scientists observed pregnant women in Germany and Austria-Hungary during World War I. Their observations seemed to show that cases of toxemia and eclampsia were cut down because of weight restriction due to food rationing during the war. The World War I "study," which was really loose observation, was taken seriously and adopted in error by many obstetricians, who prescribed a 15- to 18-pound weight-gain limit for *all* pregnant women! However, numerous later studies have shown that stringent weight gain restriction leads to low-birth-weight infants and even infant mortality and actually *causes* toxemia. Today, obstetrical practice, for the most part, limits weight gain to 20 to 25 pounds for the average woman and doctors don't worry too much if it goes to 30 pounds. Many doctors now feel that even 35 pounds and up is a reasonable weight gain for *some* women. In the case of twins, a 40- to 50-pound weight gain may not be excessive. A pregnant woman *is* eating for two—not two adults, but for herself and her baby. And pregnancy is not a time to go on a self-imposed low-calorie diet.

BIG BABIES DO NOT MEAN HARDER DELIVERIES. "If you don't stop gaining so much weight," said a nurse to Terry, a six-month-pregnant woman who had already gained twenty-two pounds, "the baby will grow too large and you'll have a difficult delivery. Take it from me. Don't gain much more or you'll be sorry when the baby starts coming." Terry became haunted by visions of a long painful labor and producing a huge baby. Fortunately, since she became dizzy and tired if she didn't eat enough, she kept right on eating plenty of good food. (See "Weight Problems," pp. 79–82.) Terry ended up gaining thirty pounds, had a six-hour labor, and produced a beautiful eight-pound two-ounce girl. But she was made unduly anxious by old wives' tales repeated by professionals who should have known better. Weight restriction may produce smaller babies, but they are not necessarily easier to deliver. Studies show that low-birth-weight babies may have more complications in delivery than normal-birth-weight babies of over five and a half pounds. When a mother is malnourished, her uterus and placenta do not grow enough. During delivery, contractions may be poor. Delivery may have to be induced and Caesarean section is often necessary.

## WHY YOUR PREGNANT BODY NEEDS . . .

PROTEIN. Have plenty (at least seventy-six grams) of protein each day for a healthy baby and a healthy, pretty you. Protein provides building blocks for the synthesis of the fetus and placenta. Your developing baby's brain is particularly in need of protein, and you need extra protein because of the increase in your total amount of blood, uterine mass, and breast tissue during pregnancy. Protein also maintains and repairs your body tissues and muscles and gives you healthy, glossy hair and pretty nails.

Sources: lean meat, fish, poultry, eggs, milk, cheese, dried beans, nuts, cereals, and fortified or whole-grain breads.

CARBOHYDRATES. Carbohydrates are found in starches and sugars. They are a major source of fuel or energy. Carbohydrates work in step with other food essentials to sustain your body and provide heat. Carbohydrates are also an important source of calories that you need to have a healthy body.

Sources: whole grain breads, cereals, fruits, vegetables. Try to use unrefined starches and sugars since their nutrient values have not been removed through processing.

# WHAT SHOULD I EAT EACH DAY?

Here is an easy way to make sure you get the proper amounts of a balanced varied diet every day. Since the body cannot store nutrients for an extended period of time, make sure you have the minimum from each group every day and even more if you feel the need for it. We've divided the required proteins, fats, and carbohydrates into simple groups with the help of nutritionist Esther Wallace of New York Hospital Clinic of Nutrition in New York City.

## Milk Group

3–4 servings of any of the following:

—Fortified whole, fat free, or skim milk (8 oz. equals one serving); or

—All cheeses (1 oz. hard cheese equals 1 serving); or

—Yogurt (8 oz. equals 1 serving)

## Meat Group

6 oz. per day or 3 servings of 2 oz. each of any of the following:

—Beef   —Fish
—Veal   —Liver (once a
—Pork     week)
—Lamb   Cut down on
—Poultry   meats with
      fats, salts,
      and added
      preserva-
      tives—espe-
      cially nitrates
      and nitrites.

## Vegetable and Fruit Group

7–8 servings (½ cup) of any of the following:

—All fruits or juices

—All vegetables or juices

Include daily at least 1 serving of foods rich in vitamin C—oranges or grapefruit—and also some rich in vitamin A—dark green or yellow vegetables.

## Bread Group

4–6 servings of any of the following:

—Rice (½ cup equals 1 serving)

—Pasta (½ cup equals 1 serving)

—Enriched whole grain bread (1 slice equals 1 serving)

—Whole grain cereals (¾ cup = 1 serving)

—Crackers (3 equals 1 serving)

## Other Foods

—Butter, margarine and oil (you can get these from fats, cheese and milk)

—Nuts and seeds

—Iodized salt

—Water and other liquids—at least 8 glasses per day

—Vitamin supplements as the doctor orders them

FATS. The popular pursuit of the fat-free diet is not a good course for nutrition during pregnancy. A moderate amount of fats is very important to an all-around balanced diet. Fats provide fatty acids which are essential for good nutrition.

Fats are also another calorie source and a source of energy. Fats are necessary for healthy skin and glossy hair. Be sure not to cut out fats entirely even if you are trying to keep your weight under control.

## SPECIAL VITAMINS AND MINERALS YOU NEED TO LOOK AND FEEL YOUR BEST FOR PREGNANCY

Most good books about nutrition during pregnancy will tell you why each vitamin and mineral is necessary for a healthy pregnancy and healthy baby. In this section we discuss the special ones which directly affect your appearance and the way you feel during pregnancy. Naturally, *all* vitamins and minerals make for an all-around healthy body. (The required amounts of each vitamin and mineral are taken from the government's Recommended Daily Dietary Allowances.)

IRON. If you're feeling generally run-down or your skin has a paleness no blusher can correct, you may have iron-deficiency anemia. This is the most common medical complaint among pregnant women and has a great deal to do with your looking and feeling good during these nine months. Other symptoms of iron-deficiency anemia are soreness of the mouth, heart palpitations after exercise, and excessive fatigue.

You need triple your usual intake of iron during pregnancy, a minimum of thirty to sixty milligrams per day. This is for your additional red blood cell production as well as for your baby's blood supply. Iron pills prescribed by your doctor are the most convenient source of iron. In addition to these pills, sources for iron are the following: beef liver, calves' liver, liverwurst, pâté, chopped chicken liver, egg yolk, dried apricots, prunes, dried beans, spinach, kale and other green vegetables, molasses, kidney, and other lean meats. Cooking in an iron skillet adds more iron to your food. When eaten along with liver or other lean meats, ascorbic acid or vitamin C (found in citrus fruits) facilitates absorption of iron by the body.

CALCIUM. If you're suffering with leg cramps during your pregnancy, too little calcium in your diet or poorly metabolized calcium may be the reason. The fetus absorbs eighty-four percent of all the calcium you eat in order to build its teeth and bones, so it is easy for you to become deficient. Your own growing needs during pregnancy also call for extra calcium (at least 1,200 milligrams). Sources of calcium are: milk (both whole and skim), cheese, yogurt, buttermilk, butter, cottage cheese, sour cream, ice cream. Vitamin D (fish and cod liver oil) can help metabolize calcium. If you are deficient in calcium your doctor may prescribe calcium tablets.

VITAMIN A. In order to keep your skin rosy and pretty during pregnancy, your eyes functioning properly, help ward off infection, and serve the needs of your growing baby, you will need to take in at least 1,000 milligrams of vitamin A each day. Foods rich in vitamin A are: dark green leafy vegetables, whole milk, butter, margarine, eggs, yellow fruits and vegetables.

VITAMIN C. This vitamin helps bind cells together, build collagen, and strengthen capillaries which are under stress during pregnancy. When you don't have enough vitamin C your system is weakened and you bleed easily. When you brush your teeth during pregnancy your gums may bleed, and increasing your vitamin C intake may remedy this. A minimum of sixty milligrams per day is recommended. Lack of vitamin C can cause a smaller uterus and a more difficult labor. Vitamin C also helps fight infection. Sources of this vitamin are: citrus fruits, berries, bananas, vegetables such as broccoli, green peppers, tomatoes, and white potatoes.

Other important vitamins and minerals essential for looking and feeling good during pregnancy include *vitamin D* found in enriched milk, the *B vitamins* (including the very important folic acid), and *phosphorus* found in fruits, meats, dairy products, vegetables, and whole-grain breads and cereals.

VITAMIN-MINERAL SUPPLEMENTS. As an aid to both your health and beauty, the special pregnancy or prenatal vitamins provide all or some of the recommended daily allowances of vitamins A, D, E, C, folic acid, thiamin, riboflavin, niacinamide, $B_6$, $B_{12}$, and minerals calcium, iodine, iron, and magnesium, as a supplement to your food.

Don't let vitamin pills give you a false sense of security. Vitamins cannot supply protein, calories, or energy—the most important elements of nutrition for a pregnant woman. If you tend to let vitamins replace a meal, you might be better off dropping the vitamins and eating a good meal so that you get the right nutrients. Vitamin pills should be used only on doctor's orders. Never take megadoses of vitamins since they can be very harmful.

SALT TALKS (SODIUM). Medical ideas about certain subjects change at a discomfortingly rapid pace—and salt, or sodium, is one of those topics. The controversy surrounding the intake of salt during pregnancy leaves one feeling very insecure about the accuracy of medical science.

At the beginning of this century, salt was thought to contribute to toxemia. Salt restriction was the command for every pregnant woman. These beliefs have now been superseded by new research. The National Academy of Sciences in its booklet *Recommended Dietary Allowances* states, "It is difficult to justify dietary sodium limitation in healthy women during pregnancy on the basis of either animal or clinical evidence." Sodium is an essential mineral. It regulates body fluid volume. Women who are pregnant have an even greater need for sodium since their maternal and fetal tissues are growing. The typical diet does contain adequate amounts of salt. Salt your food to taste unless you tend to heavily salt your foods. Moderation is a good rule of thumb.

Most obstetricians now believe that there is no need to restrict your salt unless you develop edema or other medical complications. If these complications occur, your doctor will advise. A few doctors still believe that salt should be restricted throughout pregnancy. Talk to your obstetrician about his ideas. If your doctor limits your salt intake be especially careful of any drugs or antacids containing sodium bicarbonate.

Diuretics, the water reducing medication, should *never* be taken without your doctor's approval. Diuretics are not administered as freely during pregnancy as they were years ago because—paradoxically—they may bring on toxemia. Doctors give them when necessary to treat very serious medical conditions.

## WEIGHT PROBLEMS

"HELP, I'M BALLOONING." Why do women gain weight so differently during their pregnancies? One woman we interviewed gained 10 pounds and another we interviewed gained 70. The total weight gain for most women during pregnancy is somewhere in between. Pregnancy books present charts which explain why you should gain a total of 24 pounds—fetal tissues, 7½ pounds; placenta, 1 pound; amniotic fluid, 2 pounds; uterus growth, 2 pounds; breast growth, 1½ pounds; and increase in blood, 3½ pounds. The remaining 6½ pounds is made up of stored body fat and tissue fluid.

These extra amounts of stored body fats and tissue fluid are the great variables in pregnancy. The pregnant body can store up to 20 pounds of water without running into such medical problems as edema and toxemia. As for stored fat, the government's Committee on Maternal Nutrition reports that when you become pregnant, the body resets its internal mechanism to stimulate fat storage, i.e., you gain weight. When you have your baby, this mechanism reverts to its prepregnancy level. (The Committee's report is listed in the Bibliography at the back of the book.)

"I'M CONSTANTLY STARVING." Pregnancy and its hormones can have a field day with your appetite. During the first trimester you may feel nauseated, fatigued, and lose your appetite. Or you may feel like eating all the time to quell the nausea, compensate for your lack of energy, or simply because you desire food.

Any time from your first month on you may feel ravenous. The "I'm hungry all the time" syndrome has its basis in the endocrinological changes of pregnancy. Hormones cause the blood sugar levels to fluctuate to greater extremes and thereby cause hunger more frequently. Eating small meals throughout the day can help remedy this problem.

Your taste buds actually go through a physiological change during pregnancy. Everything may taste wonderful and you may develop cravings for sweets or salty foods such as pretzels, and, yes, pickles. You may develop such aversions that a pot of perking coffee or a lit cigarette will make you flee from the room. Listen to your body. Nature gives pregnant women radar against possible harmful substances.

The big problem most women experience during pregnancy is differentiating between desire for food as a bodily need and desire for food as a consolation for depression or anxiety. Women who tend to gain excessive weight while pregnant have the same problem when they're not pregnant. Pregnancy *does* change your life-style and the hormones of pregnancy do make you moody, stimulating the desire to eat for comfort rather than nourishment. During pregnancy we tend to pamper ourselves so we overindulge cravings for foods. Some women are so excited and anxious to show the world they are pregnant that they stuff themselves to "look" pregnant. When they reach the ninth month, they find that this does not pay off.

How much should you gain each month? Charlotte's obstetrician told her in one of his practiced, routine, prenatal-care lectures, "about two and a half pounds per month. This means that if there are nine months of pregnancy, nine times two and a half equals twenty-two and a half pounds in all." This advice is rather simplistic. Very few women will gain the same amount of weight each month. Your appetite may be turned on or off by nausea during the first trimester. During the second trimester, when most women feel pretty well, metabolism is speeded up and appetite will probably increase. This also is variable. The third trimester is a notorious weight gain period because the baby is growing rapidly. However, some women report they can't finish their meals because the baby is pressing up against their stomach. The variation in weight gain patterns was astounding among the women we talked to.

As we said in the beginning of the chapter, the trick is to eat a well-balanced and varied diet. *Don't* indulge all your cravings—especially when they're for chocolate and root beer. Your weight is one of the few variables you can—to some degree—control.

It's not up to your doctor to police your eating habits. Many mothers we talked to starved themselves the day before their checkups. Many pregnant women wind up in the obstetrician's waiting room in light cotton dresses and canvas shoes in the dead of winter for the lightest weigh-in possible. Eat well for yourself and your baby—not your doctor!

If you are eating properly and are still gaining a lot of weight, discuss it with your obstetrician. Outline exactly what you're eating. You may have a medical problem.

"I WAS HEAVY WHEN I GOT PREGNANT." What if you're overweight to begin with? As we stated before, pregnancy is not the time to diet. In years past overweight women were told that pregnancy was a good time to lose weight. If they gained *no* weight during pregnancy, they would automatically be fifteen pounds lighter when they gave birth. Today we know this is a dangerous practice. Overweight women need to supply their own bodies and that of their babies with all the necessary nutrients every day. Studies show that heavier women tend to gain water weight during pregnancy while underweight women tend to gain fat.

Now is the time to teach yourself new nutrition habits. Write down everything you eat and check with our sample menus and minimum daily requirements chart. You probably know that you shouldn't be eating empty calories during this important nutritional time. Eat carefully but well now and knuckle down to a good reducing diet (such as Weight Watchers) *after* you have had your baby and have stopped breast-feeding.

"I'M UNDERWEIGHT—HOW MUCH SHOULD I GAIN?" If you're underweight to begin with, you ought to gain more weight than the average woman. You may be able now to make up the weight for your own body as well as for your baby. Often pregnancy gives you a wonderful appetite and your problem is solved. Many underweight women, however, have food avoidance habits built into their lives. Try to take it easy, rest and relax to improve your appetite. Schedule six meals a day and stick to them. Do all the things those with weight problems try not to do. Enjoy healthy desserts, have cream with coffee or cereal, butter your bread, eat high-calorie foods such as milkshakes, nuts, cheese. Eat your food slowly and with relish.

## EATING FOR RELIEF—DIETARY REMEDIES FOR COMMON PROBLEMS

Besides weight loss or gain and proper nutrition, you may have other dietary concerns during pregnancy. No one feels beautiful when she has physical problems—especially gastrointestinal ones or others that keep her running to the bathroom. Here are some common ailments that the right kinds of food can help.

NAUSEA. Nausea, morning sickness, and vomiting are energy-sapping and can be the most overriding discomfort of pregnancy. Nausea usually ends after the first trimester but sometimes continues all the way through the nine months. If you are sick in the morning, try the old trick of eating salted crackers. Have them waiting on your night table to eat in bed before getting up. For nausea that continues all day long, eat frequently to keep your stomach full. Eat a little bit every hour if you can. Carry crackers or fruit with you for tense moments. Avoid fatty, spicy, and gassy foods. Eat a high protein snack before going to sleep at night so your stomach won't be empty and subject to nausea in the morning. Protein takes longer than carbohydrates to digest.

One trick we've heard of is to eat some of your meals dry—a piece of toast or cereal without milk. Avoid beverages with these dry meals. Try to drink beverages (iced are best) by themselves, since fluids mixed with solids often aggravate nausea. Get lots of fresh air and ventilate your apartment or home thoroughly. If your nausea is bad, please notify your doctor. He may prescribe antinausea medication in severe cases.

Here are some foods the women we interviewed found helpful in quelling nausea:

Sweet carbonated beverages—especially colas—in limited amounts
Fruit juices
Peppermint tea
Yogurt
Protein foods such as eggs, milk, or meat
Popcorn
Saltines
Caramel corn
Toast with honey (no butter)


INCREASED SALIVATION (MOUTH WATERING). Excessive salivation often accompanies the nausea of early pregnancy. It is very uncomfortable, as it is difficult to swallow excess saliva and it often must be expectorated. It is worst in early pregnancy, improves in the latter half, and disappears after birth. Try chewing gum or mints and eating small meals instead of three large ones.


HEARTBURN. "My mother complained about heartburn endlessly when she was pregnant," said one new mother. "I had no idea what she was talking about—it sounded like her heart was inflamed. Then I got pregnant. Now I know. It's the thing I hated most about pregnancy."

Heartburn usually acts up in the last three months of pregnancy, but can occur at any time. It feels like a burning pain at the bottom of the rib cage near the heart, but it has nothing to do with your heart. Heartburn is caused by three different factors occurring during pregnancy: 1) the general slowing of the workings of the digestive system; 2) the baby pressing up against the stomach; and 3) the stomach acids that are reversed up into the lower part of the esophagus, burning the esophagus and causing heartburn. Heartburn is often accompanied by belching and a sour taste caused by the stomach acids.

Avoid fatty or rich foods such as bacon, mayonnaise, and french fries while suffering from heartburn. These foods are difficult to digest. Eat small meals frequently during the day rather than three large meals. Eat slowly to aid your stomach in digestion. Yogurt added to your diet is a great digestive aid. Avoid a heavy meal late in the day. Try getting up and walking about when heartburn strikes. Don't swig antacids or bicarbonate of soda since these contain amounts of sodium that can cause problems. If your heartburn is very uncomfortable, ask your doctor for advice.

CONSTIPATION. Constipation often accompanies pregnancy. Those who never had constipation before might have it during pregnancy; those prone to it before pregnancy may find it worse. Constipation results from sluggishness of the intestinal tract and abdominal muscles during pregnancy. The pressure of the baby on the bowel also contributes to the problem.

To remedy constipation, try to establish regular eliminating patterns. Avoid sitting on the toilet for prolonged periods. Don't strain. If symptoms persist, ask your doctor about special laxatives for pregnant women.

Here are some natural laxatives:

> Raw fruits (especially apples) and vegetables
> Dried fruits such as prunes, figs, dates, raisins
> Tossed salad made with any variety of greens
> Coarse cereal—especially bran
> Whole grain breads
> Licorice candy

Lots and lots of fluids—at least eight glasses of water, milk, fruit juice, coffee, and tea each day are also excellent laxatives. (But watch your consumption of caffeine—see the Medical Alert on p. 92.) Here's a natural laxative drink:

> Mix:
> ⅓ cup prune juice
> ⅓ cup apricot juice
> ⅓ cup orange juice

Chill well and drink first thing in the morning.

## PREPARING YOUR FOOD

In order to pique your appetite and maintain your glowing health, try to use the freshest meats, fish, eggs, vegetables, and fruits during your pregnancy. All perishable products should be refrigerated until you are ready to use them to prevent the build-up of bacteria. Don't take chances with cracked eggs or meat that might be turning bad.

You risk problems if you eat fish, meat, or poultry that is raw or undercooked. Undercooked pork can harbor trichinosis spores and if eaten, can cause trichinosis—a dangerous disease, especially if you are pregnant. Follow pork cooking instructions carefully. Steak tartare or other raw or rare meat can harbor parasites that cause toxoplasmosis. This is a parasitic disease that has prolonged flu-like symptoms in the mother and can be transmitted to the fetus, causing abortion, premature birth, stillbirth, or severe fetal abnormalities. This condition is not common but does occur. It's also wise to avoid raw fish (often served in Japanese restaurants) since they can also carry harmful parasites.

A conservative doctor would recommend avoiding raw shellfish during pregnancy. Shellfish are sometimes carriers of the virus that causes hepatitis. Avoid raw mussels, oysters, clams, etc. even in the best restaurants. Hepatitis is a serious illness, and during pregnancy can be very debilitating and dangerous.

Meats and fish are delicious and lower in calories when they are broiled, boiled, or poached. Frying adds a lot of calories from the shortening used to grease the pan and can cause indigestion.

Keep your foods and dishes as simple as possible. Steaming or boiling vegetables for just a few minutes only conserves nutrients. Stay away from processed foods. Fancy sauces are time-consuming and contain lots of calories. Now might be a good time to experiment with herbs and other seasonings as a flavorful substitute.

In the next few pages we list a typical menu from a day in the life of Alva and Joanne, both very pregnant. We've also listed some high-energy snacks and foods to freeze in your ninth month—for easy preparation when you come home from the hospital with your brand-new baby.

"ALVA'S MENU."

Alva was a total vegetarian until she became pregnant. She then added fish and poultry to her diet for more protein. Here is a typical day's menu for this beautiful model. (Recipes for starred dishes below.)

*Breakfast* ("I divide my pregnant breakfast into two smaller meals— one when I get up and the other a few hours later.")

*First Breakfast*
*Blender fruit drink*
Cut up any fruit in season and place it into a blender. (Alva especially loves fresh apples, bananas, pineapples, and strawberries.) Add fresh plain yogurt, fresh whole milk, and one raw egg. Add molasses or honey to taste and blend.

*Second Breakfast*
*Cereal with milk* ("Wheatena with wheat germ and raw bran is one of my favorites.")
Or, if she is working, she orders *toast with tea or coffee* or some *dried mixed fruit and nuts* from a health food store. She carries them for snacks. She also has *milk or orange juice.*

*Lunch*
If she is working, Alva orders in a *soup* and *sandwich* of cheese, lettuce, tomato on whole wheat bread with mayonnaise.
At home she has *leftovers* from the evening before—*steamed vegetables* or *tuna casserole** or a *stew.* She also drinks *carrot juice* made in her juicer. ("It's brain food for the baby—I drink between eight and sixteen ounces a day.")

*Midafternoon Snack*
*Cookies with milk*
Cookies are from the health food store and are made with either granola, date, bran, and whole wheat or a combination of these. ("Quick energy.") Sometimes she has a serving of *cottage cheese.*

*Dinner* ("I like to keep dinner light—and I always have.")
*Baked shrimp**
*Baked potato*
*Salad** with Alva's dressing*
*Fresh apple juice* ("I rarely eat dessert.")


*Before Bed*
*Carrot juice* or *raspberry tea* ("It helps avoid nausea"), *sage tea* ("It calms contractions"), or *lavender tea* ("Great for insomnia")


*All Day*
"I drink lots of water all day long. Maybe ten or more glasses in all. I snack on dried fruit and nuts whenever I feel hungry."


*For Quick Energy*
A spoonful of *honey* or *blackstrap molasses* ("If I'm really dragging and tired, I just take a nap.")


*Tuna Casserole*

1 can tuna in oil (no additives)
1 chopped onion
1 chopped green pepper
1 tablespoon safflower or olive oil
Dash tamari
Fresh grated cheddar cheese
Fresh grated parmesan cheese
½ cup milk
Whole wheat noodles

Cook noodles until almost tender. Drain. Sauté onions and peppers in safflower or olive oil. Season with tamari. Poor off excess oil and add drained tuna. Mix in casserole dish with noodles, sautéed onions and peppers, milk, cheddar cheese. Top with parmesan cheese. Bake for 35 minutes without cover until top begins to brown. Serves 2.

*Baked Shrimp*

Wash, devein, and leave shells on 1½ lbs. jumbo shrimp. Grate ½
clove of garlic and mix with melted butter in a sauce pan. Arrange
shrimp on a shallow casserole dish and pour butter or soy margarine
and garlic mixture over the shrimp. Then squeeze fresh lemon on the
shrimp. Bake for 25 minutes at 350 degrees until shrimp are crispy
but still juicy. Remove shells and place under broiler for five minutes.
"They're incredibly good and moist. Perfect for a light dinner."

*Salad*

(Use as much of the following as you like)
Romaine lettuce
Watercress
Alfalfa sprouts
Tomato
Fresh mushrooms
Lightly steamed broccoli (sometimes)
Fresh peas
1 square tofu (soybean curd—a great source of protein—found in
health food stores)
Avocado

*Salad Dressing*

1 part freshly squeezed lemon
3 parts safflower or olive oil
1 clove garlic squeezed through garlic crusher
1 teaspoon dried mustard
Several dashes tamari
Fresh pepper to taste
Sea salt

Combine ingredients with wire wisk and mix into salad just before
serving.

"JOANNE'S MENU." Joanne is eight months pregnant here. She cooks for her husband and son as well as for herself. Joanne craved vegetables all through her pregnancy. "By the time the baby comes," says Joanne, "my poor family will never want to see another helping of green beans or asparagus again!"

Here's her typical day's menu:

> *Breakfast* ("In my early pregnancy I would have a
> glass of prune juice to start. Now in my eighth month I have a
> half a grapefruit and half an English muffin with butter and Gouda
> cheese and fresh coffee and milk.")
>
> If Joanne's still hungry, she has the other *half English muffin with but-*
> *ter and jam.* ("On weekends I like to cook a big breakfast for my
> family. I make pancakes or soft-boiled or poached eggs.")

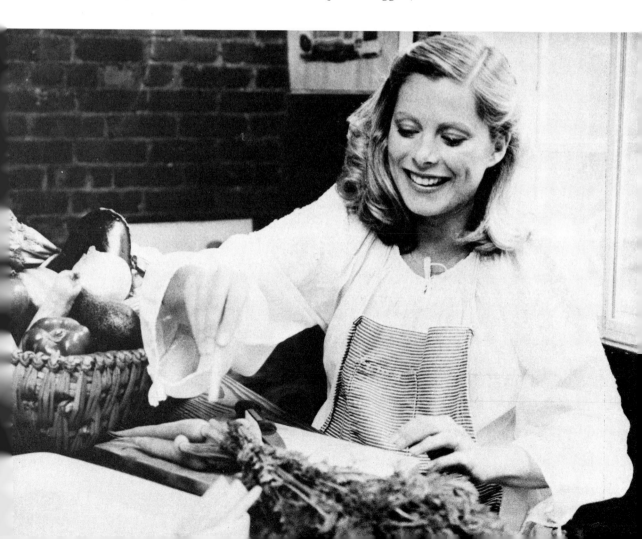

*Lunch*
*Ham and cheese sandwich on rye bread* or
*Cottage cheese with fresh fruit* or
*Bowl of raisin bran with milk*
("I eat a lot of cheese in the place of milk. I'm not crazy about milk.
My favorite cheeses are brie and French goat cheese.")

*Afternoon Snack*
*Peanut butter and jelly on rye crisp*
*Cheese on Carr's Water Biscuits*
*Tea*
("I like blander foods now in my late pregnancy. They're more
digestible.")

*Dinner*
*Chicken* or
*Fish* or
*Stir-fry beef and broccoli**
Plenty of *vegetables*
A *salad* made with lots of greens. Her favorite greens are escarole,
chicory, watercress, endives, and arugola. ("In my last trimester I just
don't feel like having a lot of potatoes and starches.")
*Ice cream* for dessert

*Evening Snack* ("I don't like to eat anything before bed—but I do
make up for it when I wake up the next morning with a big
appetite.")

*Stir-Fry Beef and Broccoli*

("My personal version of a recipe I adapted from
*The New York Times*.")

1 lb. lean flank steak
2 tbs. dry sherry
1 tsp. cornstarch
¼ cup soy sauce

1 tsp. fresh ginger (chopped fine)
1 tsp. sugar
3 whole stalks broccoli
½ tsp. salt
3 tbs. vegetable oil
¼ cup scallions
Optional: fresh snow peas, water chestnuts, mushrooms—as much as you like.

1. Slice steak at an angle into pieces ¼ thick and 2 inches long.
2. Combine sherry, cornstarch, soy sauce, ginger, and sugar in a bowl; add meat, set aside.
3. Cut broccoli florets into bite-sized pieces. Peel stalks and slice thinly. Dry with paper towel. Sprinkle salt over broccoli.
4. Heat 2 tbs. oil (or more if necessary) in a wok or heavy skillet over a high flame. Add broccoli and other vegetables, stir, and cook until tender but crisp.
5. Remove vegetables and keep warm. Add remaining oil to pan and heat. Stir in beef mixture and cook quickly until beef is cooked to desired doneness, or about two minutes.
   Add vegetables and serve. (Serves 4)

## HIGH-ENERGY SNACKS

Energy results from a well-balanced diet rather than from particular dishes. To achieve the energy you desperately need during pregnancy, you must eat enough foods from each food group to allow the body to metabolize efficiently. When metabolism is operating well, high energy results.

Although mountain climbers carry chocolate bars to eat when their energy flags, you won't need this kind of sugar jolt. Carbohydrate snacks do give quick energy, but snacks rich in protein or fats last hours longer. More wholly nutritious energy snacks are recommended. Try ours:

- Dip carrot sticks in peanut butter or creamed cheese, or spread either on one half celery stalk.

- Mix your own dried fruit-nut snacks. Combine peanuts, sunflower and pumpkin seeds, raisins, and dried fruit. Keep mixture in a small plastic bag in your purse for a surreptitious snack while working, attending a class, or on the bus ride home.
- Roll sliced ham around chunks of Swiss cheese for an easy snack.
- Keep your vegetable bin full of green and yellow vegetables. Clean carrots, zucchini, celery, and green beans. Keep them in a plastic container of water in your refrigerator for a low-calorie, high-energy snack. Mix a dip of plain yogurt and Italian dressing mix.
- There are times one cannot resist some wonderful salty junk food taste. When this urge overcomes you, pass up the pretzels and potato chips and make popcorn. Try the popcorn popper that uses hot air instead of hot oil. This saves you calories.
- Spread wedges of apple with your favorite soft cheese.
- Slice fresh strawberries into a bowl and dribble with honey. Add plain yogurt and stir gently. This treat is as delicious as a sundae and much more nutritious.

| MEDICAL ALERT | CAFFEINE |
|---|---|

A cup or two of coffee or tea each day seems to be fine for most pregnant women. However, excess amounts of caffeine found in coffee, tea, and cola, or even a little caffeine for certain women can cause headaches, insomnia, nausea, diarrhea, irregular heartbeat, and increased circulation. Caffeine quickly crosses the placenta to increase the circulation of your baby and stimulate his respiratory system. One study showed that women who drank six or more cups of coffee daily were more likely to have spontaneous abortions, stillbirths, and premature births. Cut down on coffee, tea, or cola. Some women find they must totally cut out their intake of caffeine during pregnancy.

Many people love a cocktail or two before dinner or enjoy a little wine with their meal. But these indulgences can often cause problems for both you and the baby.

Alcohol is full of carbohydrates and has no nutritive value. It quickly reaches the fetus—as a matter of fact, if a woman becomes drunk, her unborn baby becomes drunk as well.

Most of us know that drinking binges are bad for the baby but what is little known is the fact that one ounce of pure alcohol daily—especially during early pregnancy—can adversely affect the fetus.

Recent studies have questioned the advisability of even moderate intake of alcohol during pregnancy and have suggested doing without alcohol these nine months. If you do drink, limit yourself to two or three glasses of wine a day, or no more than two cocktails. Never omit protein when you are having an alcoholic beverage. See if you can cut out alcohol. If you can't cut it out completely, cut down to your minimum. Test yourself. There are lots of other delicious drinks—nonalcoholic—which can make you feel good and are much safer for you and your baby. We've noticed more and more pregnant women at cocktail parties are toasting with naturally carbonated water or plain fruit juices. Why not count yourself among this group? Your skin, figure, and health will all benefit.

## "DISHES TO MAKE AND FREEZE NOW, AND EAT LATER"

In the last few weeks of your pregnancy, spend some time making meals to freeze for your first few weeks postpartum. These dishes will be easy to defrost and heat. Your effort now will be appreciated when you're a tired new mother later. Serve these heated dishes with a salad, French bread, and cheese or butter.

*Cook and freeze:*

Any kind of stew made with beef, chicken, veal
Chili (go lightly on the chili powder if you plan to nurse)
Lasagna
Split pea or lentil soup. Accompany with sliced cold meat if you like.
Quiches. Cheese, zucchini, or shrimp quiches are easy to make and freeze if you own a food processor. Whip up the quiche mixture and pour into a frozen pie crust from the supermarket. This makes a wonderful light meal for the summer months. Serve with fruit for dessert.

Don't forget to stock up on your favorite frozen products. They're lifesavers when you have a new baby!

## WHAT TO AVOID—DRUGS, FOOD ADDITIVES, AND HOUSEHOLD DANGERS

Knowing what *not* to eat, breathe, and take, is just as important as knowing what one *should* eat during pregnancy—perhaps even more so. Although drugs and chemicals are part of our lives now, an informed pregnant woman will approach these substances as if entering a danger zone. So when in doubt—stay away—for the healthiest and most beautiful pregnancy possible.

DRUGS. Don't take *any* drugs unless your obstetrician has prescribed or approved them. Your dermatologist, allergist, dentist, or whatever specialist you see, should always speak to your obstetrician before she prescribes drugs for you while you are pregnant.

Simply because you don't need a prescription for some pills does not mean that it's all right to take them. Over-the-counter drugs can be dangerous. *All* drugs can pass through the placenta to reach your baby. The frequency and the amount of the drugs you take, their fat solubility, and your own genetic makeup determine to what extent the baby will be affected. Even when your own obstetrician prescribes drugs, discuss with him whether they are absolutely necessary. The nasal congestion or headaches characteristic of your first trimester are a common—if uncomfortable—part of pregnancy. You should consult with your doctor before trying to treat these symptoms. Obviously, if you have a raging fever or infection, you must consider your health, and that means the baby's too.

Make a list of your medications, including medicated creams and sprays as well as pills and syrup. Some women don't realize that they are taking drugs until they realize that they use an antihistamine in the morning, an aspirin in the afternoon, and a sleeping pill in the evening. All these drugs can be dangerous: antihistamines are suspected of causing birth defects; aspirin in large and frequent doses has been associated with bleeding in the newborn, miscarriage, stillbirth, and low birthweight; and sleeping pills can cause respiratory difficulties and excessive bleeding in newborns.

Other common drugs such as cough medicines, antibiotics, antinauseants, antidepressants, sex hormones, "hard" drugs, etc. have been proven to have negative effects on the growing fetus. Many drugs have not been adequately screened for their effects on pregnant women. Again—be conservative. See if you can get through that headache without medication.

FOOD ADDITIVES. Since this is your pregnancy and your precious child, exercise the best judgment at this time in limiting your food additives. Many food additives, although presently allowed on the market by the Food and Drug Administration, are under scrutiny for their possible carcinogenic effect on humans. Read the labels on food containers at the supermarket. Choose foods that say "No preservatives or artificial ingredients added." Avoid routine use of additives such as preservatives BHA and BHT (in cereals, cake mixes, etc.), certain dyes, MSG or monosodium glutamate (often found in Chinese food as well as frozen and canned foods), and nitrates and nitrites (found in cured meats and fish).

Sugar substitutes, saccharin and sorbitol, the diet aids of millions of figure-conscious women, are suspected of carcinogenicity and should be avoided during pregnancy. If you've been drinking two diet sodas every day for the last five years, drop this luxury now. Replace them with something nutritious and safe. Choose drinks such as fruit juices, milk, water. Naturally carbonated water with lime is a wonderful refresher that has no calories or additives.

Eat meats that are low in fats and make sure fish or meat is from an area that has not been contaminated. PCB (polychlorinated biphenyls), PBB (polybrominated biphenyls), mercury, and pesticide contamination in certain geographical areas and bodies of water have made many foods unsafe—especially for pregnant and lactating women. As a general rule, cut off all fat from your meats. Write to the Environmental Defense Fund, 1525 18th Street NW, Washington, D.C. 20036, for the latest information on geographical pollution.

HOUSEHOLD DANGERS. The nesting instinct is never so strong as during pregnancy. Many women we talked to were fixing up and preparing their homes for the new addition to the family. Couples and families were moving into larger apartments or houses and redoing the places themselves.

This is lots of fun, challenging, and especially fulfilling while you're pregnant. However, you should know there are risks in exposing yourself to some of the chemicals and substances used in the house. Your nose and stomach are especially sensitive to chemical odors during pregnancy and can serve as a trustworthy guide to what should be avoided. If you find that bleaching fluids turn your stomach, simply move the bleaching clothes to an area where you will not be exposed to their smell. Or have someone else do your bleaching. Take tips from your body—it's reacting physiologically to substances that normally might not bother you. These fumes can also put stress on the body's detoxifier, the liver. The liver is already overtaxed because of pregnancy, so avoid anything that smells noxious or offensive. The following substances may cause you and your unborn child everything from physical stress to fetal abnormality.

*Kitchen.*

1. Avoid fumes from: oven cleaners, bleaching agents, dyes, other cleaning agents—especially aerosol—in enclosed areas.
2. Do not use improperly glazed pottery.

*Other Rooms.*

Avoid:
1. Mothball fumes
2. Exterminating pesticides (some are suspected of having carcinogenic effects on the fetus). Avoid exterminated rooms for a few days after spraying.
3. Stay away from cats and their feces—they can carry a parasite which causes toxoplasmosis. If you already own a cat, you may be immune. A blood test will tell. The veterinarian can test your cat to see if it carries toxoplasmosis.

*Household Refinishers.*

1. Avoid fumes from:
   Interior paints (latex paints may be safe)
   Paint thinners, strippers, and solvents
   Benzine (a warning has been placed on this)
   Polyurethane
   Aerosol paints or other aerosol products
   Furniture strippers
   Contact cement
   Many glues
2. Avoid sanding dust from old interior paint (which may contain lead), putty, and plaster.
3. Avoid asbestos and fiberglass.

*Outdoors.*

1. Avoid: fertilizers, pesticides, insecticides, and herbicides. DDT is lethal. It has been banned although many people in rural sections still use it.

2. Avoid a lot of charcoal-broiled food.
3. Avoid exhaust fumes from vehicles. Check your own car to see if it is properly vented so you're not continually breathing carbon monoxide.
4. Avoid exterior paints (which contain lead).
5. Don't dig in soil where cats may have excreted their feces. Their litter may carry toxoplasmosis. (See p. 97.)

| MEDICAL ALERT | SMOKING |
| --- | --- |

It's impossible to avoid smoke-filled rooms altogether if you work and go out to restaurants. But if you and your husband don't smoke you can see to it that your home is smoke-free. If you do smoke you have probably been chided already about the damage you are doing to your own health and beauty (see p. 44). Now that another human is going to be affected by the smoking habit, the pressure on you is building.

Smoking just one cigarette will raise your carbon monoxide level by ten percent and thereby lower the amount of oxygen available to the baby. Cutting down fetal oxygenation can cause all sorts of problems for the baby. One well-known study shows that seven- to eleven-year-old children whose mothers smoked one-half a pack of cigarettes or more per day while they were pregnant had a higher mental and physical retardation rate than those whose mothers did not smoke. Nicotine also makes it harder to utilize vitamin C.

EATING SENSIBLY. "It seems all of us pregnant women will have to lock ourselves up and eat nothing but organically grown alfalfa sprouts," complained twenty-four-year-old Janet, a well-read but discouraged woman in her second month of pregnancy. Warnings about food additives and chemicals in our environment by the newspapers, TV, this and other pregnancy books *do* seem depressing.

Cheer up. You're going to be fine if you eat well and are sensible about drugs and chemicals. It's not so difficult to eat healthy foods. Think of all the ripe and juicy fruits available, the crisp green and yellow vegetables, the crunchy whole grain breads, tender lean meats, and rich homemade custards. Buy and cook the best—you and your baby deserve it.

# CHAPTER ·IV·
# Your Pregnant Body— Staying Healthy and Fit

"I HAVE INSOMNIA AT NIGHT, leg cramps in the morning, my back hurts, my feet swell, and I feel so heavy all day long," said a friend who at six months was already tired of being pregnant. "I thought pregnancy was supposed to be fun." The aches and pains as well as the unexpected bloom you enjoy while you're pregnant are all caused by the truly enormous changes that are taking place in your body during these nine months. Your new and changing shape and size will make it difficult for you to cope with old situations such as zipping up your boots and lifting your toddler. There are twinges and discomforts—such as pains in the groin, excess vaginal discharge, varicose veins, and more serious problems that need prompt medical attention. The important thing is to know what is happening to you and why, and what you can do about it. Make these nine months a time when you get in closer touch with your own body. It may not be true, as the mother of one thirty-year-old friend of ours thought, that pregnancy "refreshes" the body and gets all the female parts working. But pregnancy *is* a rite of passage, part of your own physical and psychological evolution as a woman. How you maintain your body and cope with the changes during pregnancy will have an effect on your health and beauty for the rest of your life.

*Opposite page:* Liz continues her daily jog right through pregnancy.

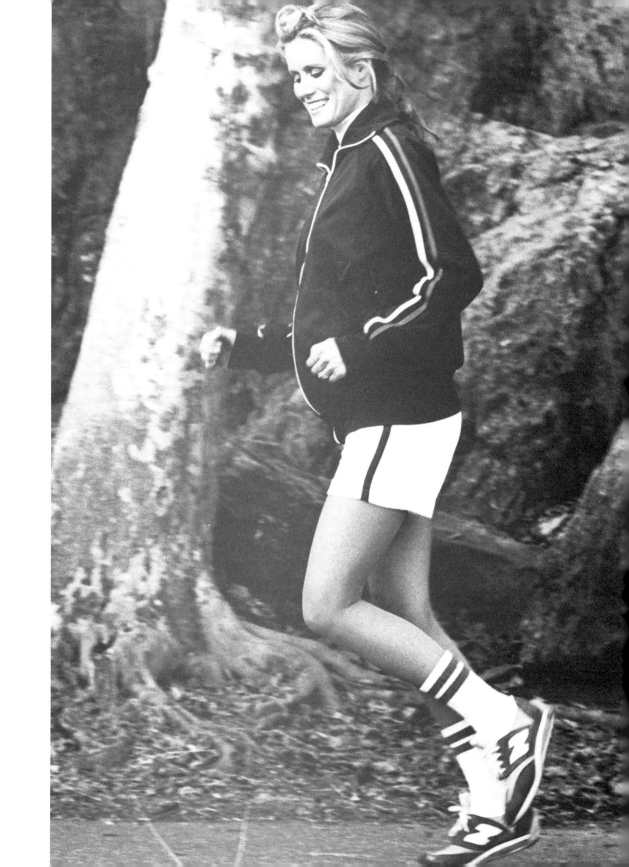

## "OH MY ACHING BACK!"—HOW TO HOLD AND MOVE YOUR BODY

What is more poetic than a pregnant woman who carries herself tall and gracefully? And what is more wincingly unattractive than a splay-footed, back-bowed woman waddling through her last months? Poor posture is not only a matter of beauty but also personal health. Bowing or arching the back, spreading the fanny, and tipping the pelvis forward all feel natural because the weight of the uterus has shifted the center of your body's gravity. But these are destructive to your sensitive back muscles, ligaments, and joint tissues—the latter weakened by pregnancy hormones—and can lead to back problems for the first time in your life.

The solution is to attempt to keep the pelvis tilted back. To feel the correct alignment put your hands on your hips and pull *back* while tucking buttocks in. (See illustration.) This prevents stretching the abdominal muscles and shortening the muscles behind. If you tilt the pelvis forward, the spine becomes curved, with the resultant backaches, flabby abdomen, and a sagging pelvic floor.

Make a conscious effort to stand and sit straight. Keep your shoulders level and pretend your body is hanging by a string. Don't stand stiffly and throw your shoulders back like a West Point cadet. Relax and keep this string effect in mind. Check to make sure you're tucking in your buttocks and pulling up your abdominal muscles. Put equal weight on both feet and don't lock your knees.

Try to kneel, stand, and sit with a straight spine. Don't wear high heels, pick up heavy objects, or move suddenly. You can also strengthen and stretch your back muscles with exercise (see pp. 132, 136) and make your abdominal muscles help take up some of the work load. But get your doctor's approval before you continue any exercises.

You may feel silly relearning how to move and walk, but with this new bulk on your body, such simple tasks as giving yourself a pedicure can be herculean. We forget how agile we were with slim tummies. Here are some solutions to three common problems: sleeping, getting out of bed, and bending and lifting.

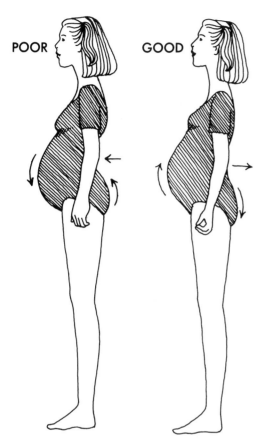

POOR  GOOD

Examples of poor (*left*) and good (*right*) posture. It's easy to let yourself fall into bad posture habits since the body's weight shifts as the baby grows.

1. If your pregnant abdomen feels uncomfortable in most sleeping positions, sleep on your side. Most pregnant women prefer the left side since the major blood vessels are on the right side of the body. Bend your upper leg and place a pillow under it.

2. Getting out of bed presents a problem in your later months of pregnancy. Springing from the bed tends to cramp previously loosened and relaxed muscles. Practice the following technique early on—it's better for your back in nonpregnant life too. Lie on your back and pull your knees up. Roll over on your side and push yourself up to a sitting position using both hands. Ease your legs over to the side of the bed and you're up!

3. Again, even when you're not pregnant, the following method of lift-

ing from the floor is advisable. To lift your child or an object, squat down, moving your pelvis close to the object. Keep your back straight, your pelvis tipped back and, with your arms, lift the object straight up using your thigh muscles. The strain is then on your legs rather than your back and arms. And of course don't lift heavy objects while you're pregnant—the risk of pulling a muscle is too great.

## ABDOMINAL MUSCLES—YOUR SUPPORT SYSTEM

The most obvious change in your musculature is in front of you: in your abdominal muscles, which do one of the roughest jobs during pregnancy. They are stretched over the uterus to support the weight and bulk of the baby and water. As mentioned above, your abdominal muscles also help support your back, especially in light of the new shift of balance.

Women "show" or "pop" their abdomens at widely varying times—some show at two months and others don't pop until six. With subsequent pregnancies, you'll probably show sooner even though you may gain the same amount of weight. After the first baby, the abdominal muscles relax to a degree. "Showing" doesn't indicate anything significant about the strength of your abdominal muscles. But well-exercised abdominal muscles do make a difference after birth.

Years ago doctors reported a strange phenomenon among unmarried pregnant women. They noticed that the stomachs of these women were particularly flat and taut after delivery. Why? They practiced holding in their stomachs in an attempt not to show they were pregnant and consequently their abdominal muscles became very strong. Many pregnant women today are afraid they will hurt the baby or themselves if they pull in their stomachs. On the contrary, strengthening these muscles is extremely important during pregnancy.

"If I'd known how flabby my abdomen would be after I had the baby," said the mother of a seven-month-old, "I would have started exercises as soon as I heard I was pregnant. Even with my postpartum exercise regime,

I'm not back to my old self." A loose abdomen—after the baby is born—is the most common figure problem women experience. Some extra bulk on the abdomen is inevitable right after the baby is born. The layer of tissue that is not really flab but simply extra tissue will be reabsorbed within a few months postpartum. But the rest of the abdominal fat is from stretched abdominal muscles and perhaps extra weight gained during pregnancy. Under the influence of pregnancy hormones, abdominal muscles may become permanently stretched. Your recovery is speeded and your pregnancy is aided by good posture and exercise of the abdomen during pregnancy. (See special exercises on pp. 132–36.)

| PAINS DOWN THE SIDES OF THE ABDOMEN AND THE GROIN | MEDICAL ALERT |
|---|---|

Candy, a four-and-a-half-month pregnant lawyer, had to jump up from a conference table during a meeting. She was experiencing pains in her groin. "This is it," she thought to herself. "I'm in trouble. Something's wrong with the baby."

Her doctor quickly reassured her. Pains in the groin and pains at the sides of the abdomen usually result from the stretching of the round ligaments which hold the uterus in place. These are "growing pains" that are unique to these ligaments. The uterus, in contrast, usually grows with ease and more rapidly than the ligaments. Talk to your doctor about such pains. They are usually not cause for concern.

## UNDER PRESSURE: THE FEET AND LEGS

FEET. Feet have so much weight to carry—especially during pregnancy—it's amazing that they function as well as they do. Your feet may get very tired during pregnancy. Podiatrists also report that women develop fallen arches during pregnancy. This is an orthopedic problem and may need to be treated by a specialist. When arches fall, feet can widen and often do not return to prepregnancy size. Bunions and foot spurs can also occur if swollen feet make your shoes too tight. Stay aware of the fit of your shoes. If they are too tight, invest in a low-heeled pair of shoes in the next larger size to save your feet. (See exercises on p. 139 and Chapters I and V.)

LEGS. The extra weight of the uterus puts increased pressure on the leg veins. Blood can pool in the veins, contributing to varicosities. Water tends to collect in the feet, ankles, and legs. Rest and elevate your legs as often as possible for these problems. Leg cramps develop for a number of reasons: some doctors believe the *lack* of calcium is at fault while others believe that *too much* calcium overloads the body with phosphates and is the real culprit in the leg cramps. Other medical experts admit they don't know why these muscle spasms occur. Your leg cramps can be helped by exercises. You can also try this trick to relieve soreness in the calves caused by leg cramps. Sit on the side of your bathtub and put your legs under the faucet. Run hot water for a minute and then switch to cold water for a minute. Keep alternating the two temperatures until the soreness is gone.

VARICOSE VEINS. As the fluids and pressure build up in your body, you may develop varicose veins—a minor nuisance, a potential health problem, and downright ugly as well. If you don't have varicose veins yet, but they run in your family, do your best to prevent them by following the suggestions in this section.

Varicose veins can range from a few raised bluish vessels undulating under your skin—unsightly, but not a major problem—to the angiectids, or protruding clumps of blue-purple vessels, which are painful and energy-sapping because they limit your daily activities. They may even require surgery.

Fortunately, most varicose veins developed during pregnancy disappear after your baby is born. But the veins themselves are weakened by the varicosity, and when subsequent pregnancies place additional pressure on them, they tend to come back more severely than before. What can you do to avoid them, or keep them under control and cover them up if they *do* appear?

- Don't indulge in empty calories. They will make you gain extra pounds that put a great strain on the cardiovascular system.
- Get plenty of exercise. It promotes good circulation, and the contraction of your muscles that takes place when you exercise will help pump blood out of your legs and back to your heart.
- If you have to sit for long periods at work, force yourself to get up and move around. While you're sitting, point your toes and make circles in the air—you'll look nervous but you will be keeping blood circulating well. Don't cross your legs at the knee, but keep them slightly bent when you sit.
- At work or at home during the day, sit down and prop your feet up to chest level on a hassock or chair or whatever you can find. This reduces the pressure of blood in the veins in your legs. It feels good too.
- Support stockings are a great aid for those with varicose veins. Wear these stockings during all your waking hours—it's very important to support the veins in your legs. For most women the sheer support pantyhose works fine, and are much prettier than the heavier support hose; but if your veins are very bad you may have to wear heavy support pantyhose or hose specially fitted to your leg. Pull on your stockings before you get out of bed in the morning so your veins won't have a chance to fill up. Or, after you've showered get back into bed to rest for five minutes before putting on your stockings. Avoid knee socks and knee-high stockings even if your varicose veins are slight—they can cut off circulation. Don't wear disco-style high heels or very flat shoes. An inch to an inch-and-a-half heel is ideal.
- For the last trimester, try to sleep on your left side so the blood can circulate freely to the heart.
- There are excellent concealing makeups that can be used to cover varicose veins on the leg. COVERMARK by Lydia O'Leary works very well. You can also try wearing pantyhose a shade darker. This will help hide the discoloration and make your legs look slimmer too!

Alva's dance class combines yoga and dance. It teaches grace and agility in movement. She attends class three or four times a week for an hour. If you enjoy doing yoga, certain exercises are wonderful and relaxing but others should not be done during pregnancy. Check with a pregnancy yoga or exercise book and your doctor.

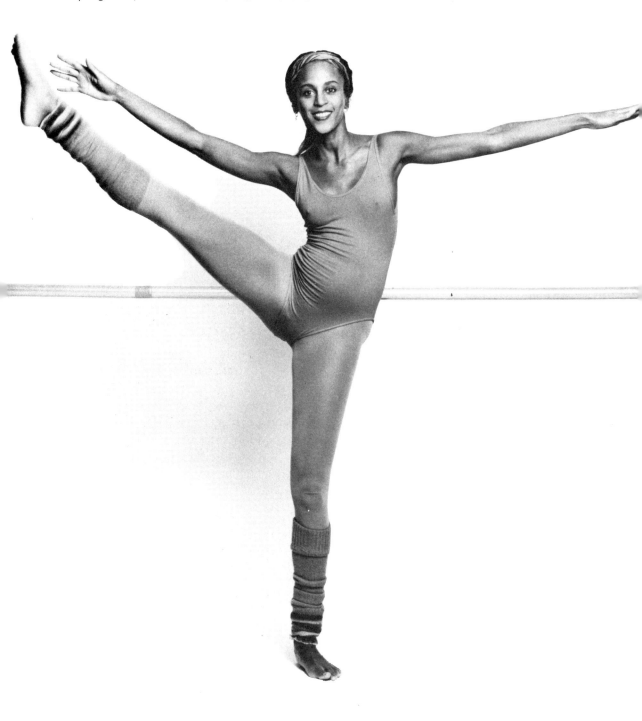

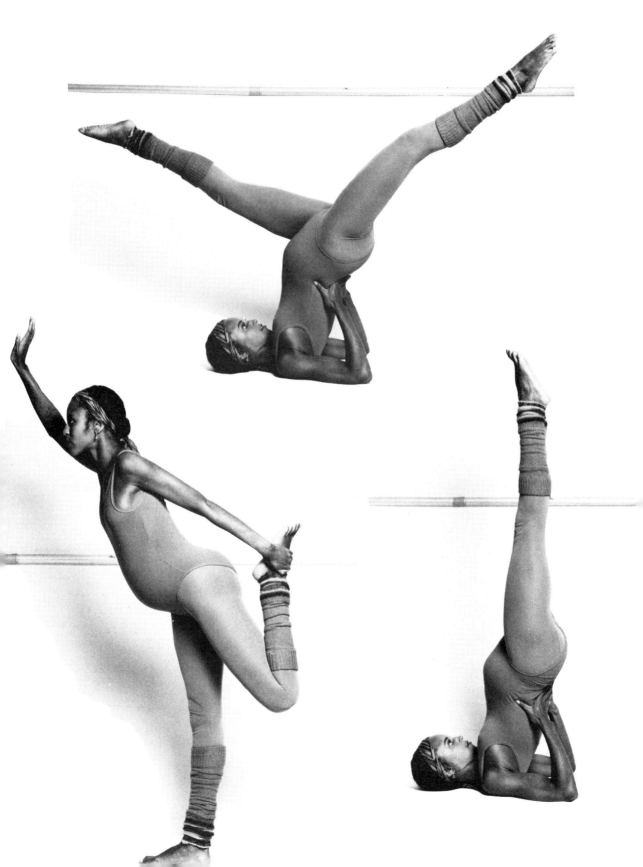

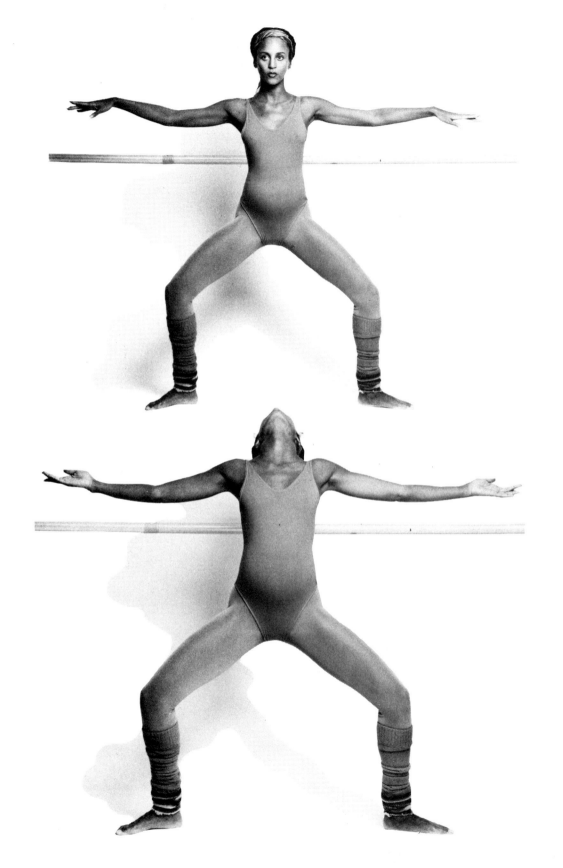

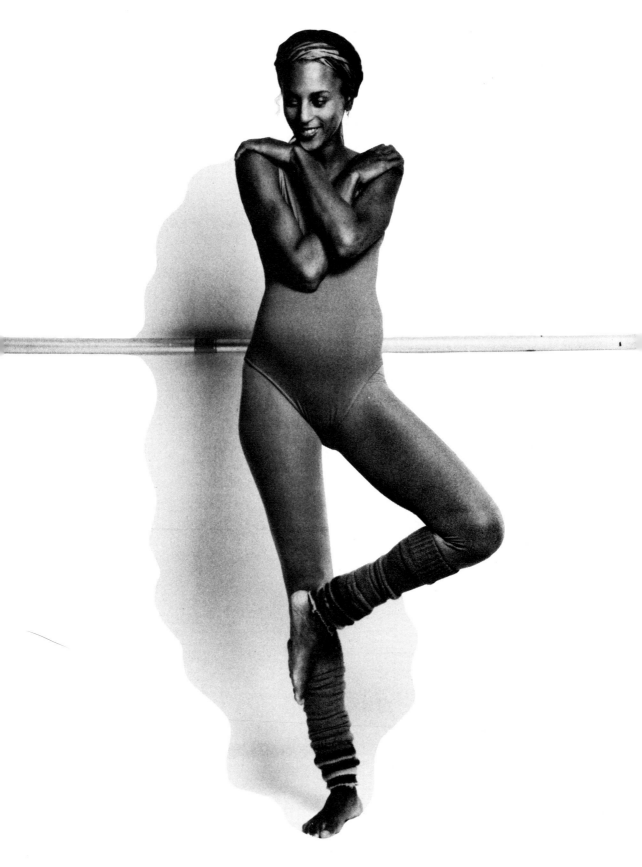

## THE SPREADING FANNY AND HEAVY THIGH SYNDROME

"The most distressing experience of pregnancy was going to half-sizes in pants," said a friend with a six-month-old baby. "My hips just outgrew the maternity size fourteens, and I wound up in the half sizes' maternity department."

Oh the eternal fanny and thigh weight problem! So many of us tend to gain weight in the fanny and thighs even when we're not pregnant. The extra pounds gained during pregnancy find their happy home in the same place. Extra weight should be reabsorbed within three to five months after delivery—unless you indulged in a lot of extra calories during pregnancy. The remaining fat is hard to lose.

The spreading fanny and heavy thigh syndrome is worsened by pregnancy hormones and/or the poor posture of bowing the back and spreading buttocks and thighs outward. Proper posture and exercise strengthen these leg, hip, and buttock muscles to help them support your extra weight. For exercises working on the hip, thigh, and buttock area see pp. 135, 137, and 140.

## HOW TO CARE FOR YOUR CHANGING BREASTS

During pregnancy, your breasts go through great changes. One of the first things you may feel is a tenderness in your breasts caused by increased vascularity and rapid growth. Your breasts sometimes continue to grow up to two sizes larger than your normal size. Due to the enriched and enlarged blood supply to your breasts, blue veins may show through your skin. These will remain visible until you stop nursing. If you don't nurse they will disappear within a month after you have your baby. The nipples and areolas will probably darken. By your fourth month your nipples will be secreting colostrum, a yellowish sticky substance rich in the nutrients and antibodies newborn babies need. You won't stop secreting it until three days after delivery, when your milk begins. Your areolas may develop little bumps called tubercles of Montgomery—small roundish elevations caused by enlarged sebaceous glands. (Their medical discoverer, Montgomery, poetically described them as "a constellation of miniature nipples scattered over a Milky Way.") They recede after pregnancy and lactation.

The most common and obvious change in your breasts is the increase in their size. Most women are thrilled. "Since the time I was a teenager I have always wanted a big bust, and now I have it," said Virginia, a pretty blonde public relations writer, five months pregnant. "I guess it's just psychological on my part, but I feel like a sex symbol—and it's fun!" Most husbands will respond to such new charms with lots of attention.

Maintaining the beauty of your breasts requires a little extra effort during pregnancy. Since most changes in the look of the breast such as stretch marks or loss of shape are thought to occur during pregnancy and not during breast-feeding, you should pamper your breasts from the beginning. Some changes can't be helped, but others are definitely preventable with a good bra and proper care.

Continue to wash your breasts as you normally do, except for soaping. Use very little soap or eliminate it entirely—since your breasts and nipples need their skin oils at this time to prevent cracking and dryness while they are growing and tender. You may find that secreted colostrum often dries on the tips of your nipples. During your bath or shower, simply use a washcloth to clean this crusting. Some doctors advise gently expressing—or gently squeezing—this colostrum a few weeks before you deliver to open the milk ducts and ease the flow of milk. Ask your obstetrician for advice and a demonstration of this exercise.

After your bath, use a pure lanolin cream on the areolas and the sides of the nipple. To allow the tips of the nipples to secrete colostrum freely, avoid covering the duct openings. You can buy small amounts of inexpensive pure lanolin from your druggist. After applying the lanolin, moisturize your entire chest area, using your favorite body lotion. Draw your hands upward from your tummy to your breast. Give yourself a delicious massage by gently encircling the breasts and spreading the moisturizer over your skin, always in an upward direction. Your skin will tingle and feel refreshed.

After the massage, expose your breasts to the air for a while. Do this whenever possible. Air is soothing if your nipples are tender and can help toughen them if you plan to nurse. (Redheads or those with fair complexions are particularly susceptible to sore nipples.) Many women buy nursing bras during their pregnancy and wear them with the flap open to expose their nipples to the air, or they cut out holes in their regular bras and wear them under clothes. The gentle friction of the clothes (don't wear burlap!) helps toughen up tender nipples and prepares them for hungry babies.

Many doctors recommend this nipple-toughening exercise for nursing mothers-to-be: Gently roll the nipple between the thumb and forefinger a few times a day; if your nipples begin to get sore, stop and resume this exercise the next day. (Some doctors feel that no exercise is needed, so ask yours.) Inverted nipples, which point inward instead of out, or flat nipples that don't protrude, might need a special exercise. Talk to your doctor if you think your nipples are inverted and ask what to do about them.

Choose a bra (nursing, pregnancy, or regular) with good support. When your breasts start to feel heavy, wear it twenty-four hours a day. Our experience and that of our friends has been that wearing a bra twenty-four hours a day helps keep the breasts firm and uplifted. The combination of a high estrogen level weakening the collagen and the physical weight of the breasts make good support a must. Your bra should be pure cotton or a cotton and polyester blend to allow air circulation and to absorb perspiration as well.

## THE GENITAL AREA

As your pregnancy progresses, the area extending from the urethra to the vagina to the rectum is also changing. The skin in this area is darkening, the labial tissues swell, and the vagina secretes more discharge.

Care of this area is simple. Since pregnancy is a time to take extra care and avoid vaginal infection, cleanliness is a must. Bathe or shower daily. To keep genitals clean, use a soft washcloth and a little soap, making sure you cleanse in the folds of the labia. When washing (or wiping after a bowel movement), start at the front of the body and wipe towards the back. Don't wash too much—that causes problems too.

Don't douche while you are pregnant. Douching isn't necessary even when you're not pregnant—except if your doctor instructs you to, of course—because the vagina is self-cleansing. When your perineal tissues are swollen, more vasuclar, and changed by the hormones of pregnancy, the skin is especially sensitive. If you introduce irritants such as perfumes or other ingredients in the commercial douche—even water—you could get rid of all the good bacteria and upset the ecology of the vagina. This may cause itching or even infection. Don't use vaginal deodorant sprays while you are pregnant. Avoid using perfume, perfumed dusting powder, or other products designed to deodorize the vaginal area.

EXCESSIVE VAGINAL DISCHARGE. Some women have made the mistake of douching or using a vaginal deodorant when they noticed excess vaginal discharge during pregnancy. This thick yellow-white leukorrhea becomes more noticeable around the fourth month, and it can make you feel less than beautiful since if often irritates the skin or the genital area and may mat your pubic hairs.

But as messy and irritating as it is, the discharge is actually cleansing your vagina and keeping it free of infection, as well as lubricating the tissues of the vagina as they become thicker, softer, and more elastic in preparation for birth. During subsequent pregnancies you may have very little discharge.

What steps can you take to feel better?

- You can wear the best invention since the wheel—an adhesive mini-pad or panty-shield. Change these as often as you need to.
- Cotton underpants are also recommended since nylon underwear doesn't breathe as well, compounding your problem by retaining heat in the genital area.
- If the vaginal tissues are irritated from the discharge, take a warm bath with one-half cup of salt added. The salt acts to soothe and restore the skin's natural ecology, like salt tears. Spread your legs to allow the water to reach inside the folds of the labia and use your finger to circulate the salt water in your vagina. If this discharge stings, itches, or burns, talk to your obstetrician.

If white cottage-cheese-like curds are noticed along with this discharge, you may have a yeast infection, a common affliction among pregnant women. Notify your doctor. He will probably prescribe an antifungal agent. The salt bath mentioned above will also help.

VARICOSE VEINS OF THE VULVA. Not all varicose veins appear in the legs. Pat, a thirty-two-year-old woman carrying her second child, was alarmed when she noticed a swelling around the opening of her vagina. Her doctor informed her she had developed varicose veins in the vulva because of the pressure on her lower abdomen by the baby and these veins would probably recede after delivery. Varicosities like this usually occur after several pregnancies since the first baby has stretched the abdominal muscles and caused the second to ride lower and create even more pressure. Your doctor may advise you to wear a maternity girdle as a treatment and a preventive.

FREQUENT URINATION, INCONTINENCE, AND CONSTIPATION. "Not only did I have to get up twice a night to go to the bathroom, but every time I sneezed or laughed hard—you guessed it—I wet my pants," said a new mother. "In the last trimester I would sometimes wear minipads for this problem. I'm so glad to hear lots of other women had these complaints too."

Chances are that one of the first signs that told you you were pregnant was that you had to urinate more frequently than before. In the first three months of your pregnancy, your expanding uterus presses against your bladder, which is located right in front of the uterus. The urge to urinate is felt often even if you have nothing to void. In the fourth month, the uterus moves up and you feel better. Then in the last months, the uterus moves down again to press against the bladder. Sometimes you can't keep a little urine from escaping when you sneeze, cough, run, or exercise. The frequent-urination problem gets better after you have your baby; but your inability to control urine—or incontinence—sometimes continues for a number of months afterward.

During and after pregnancy Kegel or pelvic floor exercises can help incontinence (see pp. 118–20). For frequent urination some doctors recommend cutting out liquids after dinner. However, denying liquids to your thirsty pregnant body might be unwise. Try to bear with the troublesome trips to the bathroom. Don't put off the urge to urinate, which could make it difficult to start urinating when you eventually decide to go. If there is any burning sensation when you urinate, let your obstetrician know immediately.

Paradoxically, while you must urinate more frequently, you may also suffer from constipation. Because the pregnant body is so thirsty for fluids and the water metabolism is so high, the body tries to extract water from every source it can—including the colon. The stools then become hard and dry, you may feel bloated, and you may experience abdominal pain. See p. 84 for more information about constipation. This constipation of pregnancy is a signal that you must increase your water intake.

PREGNANCY'S THORN: HEMORRHOIDS. "Why didn't anyone tell me about hemorrhoids?" wailed many of the mothers we talked to. Most pregnancy books and childbirth classes *don't* warn women of the great possibility that they will develop hemorrhoids—but eighty percent of all women do. You will recognize hemorrhoids (actually swollen veins) as fleshy masses protruding from the anus. They occasionally bleed after a difficult bowel movement.

You might develop hemorrhoids for a number of reasons. As your pregnancy progresses, the pressure within your veins increases with your increasing blood volume, and the uterus bears down harder on the venous system in the lower part of your body. This strain, or the effects of constipation, or the effort of birth itself, can cause hemorrhoids. Often the hemorrhoids will disappear or recede within three months after you give birth.

The tendency to develop hemorrhoids is inherited. It may not be much consolation—but you might have gotten them at a later age if pregnancy hadn't moved them up on your life schedule. To keep the problem under control and relieve the discomfort, try the following:

- Drink at least two quarts of fluids a day—especially water—to aid your digestive system.

- Eat plenty of fruits, vegetables, and bran products to keep your stools soft. Ask your doctor for a mild stool softener if your constipation is severe. Don't take a laxative without your doctor's advice.
- Commercial medications work well to relieve the itching and soreness of hemorrhoids and help in shrinking the veins.
- While taking a bath or shower, use your finger to push the swollen veins back into the rectum. This will help the healing. After a bowel movement use petroleum jelly on your finger to push the veins back inside.
- If your hemorrhoids bleed, tell your obstetrician. In the meantime, you can lie down, place a pillow under your pelvis and use balls of cotton to apply iced witch hazel to the hemorrhoids. This should help shrink them and relieve the irritation. Surgery for hemorrhoids is usually not performed until well after delivery of the last child you intend to have. (See Chapter VIII, "Your Body Postpartum.")

| MEDICAL ALERT | HERPES SIMPLEX (TYPE II) |
| --- | --- |

This venereal disease is becoming more widespread. If you have had any vaginal herpes simplex in the past or have developed any of the characteristic vaginal lesions or fever blisters during pregnancy, inform your obstetrician. If your baby comes in contact with the sores during delivery, the results are fatal in sixty percent of the cases. The babies who do live may have major neurological defects. A Caesarean section delivery is usually advised in the presence of active herpes. But most times herpes will become inactive long before you go into labor.

## PELVIC FLOOR OR KEGEL EXERCISES

One of the best things you can do to help control incontinence and relieve pressure in the pelvic area is pelvic floor or Kegel exercises developed by Dr. Arnold Kegel, a gynecologist who has devoted much research to this neglected musculature. The pelvic floor, or muscle layers supporting the pelvic organs, begins in the area around the urethra sphincter, continues to the vagina, and ends at the rectal sphincter. You can imagine how much stress these muscles experience during pregnancy under the weight and pressure of the uterus. This pressure of the uterus slows blood circulation; and since the hormones of pregnancy are softening the tissues and rendering them even weaker, the whole area is predisposed to such vascular problems as hemorrhoids and varicose veins of the vulva.

Kegel exercises help to prevent these problems—as well as others, such as prolapsing of the uterus (a condition in which the pelvic organs descend into the vagina). They teach you how to relax your pelvic muscles during delivery, thereby easing the descent of the baby down the vagina. (You'll probably learn all about this in your prepared-childbirth class.)

Another delightful benefit of Kegel exercises is the creation of new dimensions in lovemaking. One of the best places to practice is in bed, where your partner will let you know how proficient you've become. Once you gain control of the vaginal muscles, you'll learn how to control the pressure on his penis with your vaginal muscles to increase both his and your sexual pleasure. (See Chapter VI, "Sex and Pregnancy.")

HOW TO DO KEGEL EXERCISES. At first almost everyone has difficulty differentiating between the muscles of the inner thigh, buttock, and abdomen, and the pelvic floor muscles. You soon learn. Try these for starters:

1. Pretend you're urinating. Try to stop. Move the constricting effort to the vagina. Move to the rectal sphincter and pretend you're stopping a bowel movement. Now, try all these movements together, contracting, lifting up, counting to five, and letting down to the count of five.
2. Practice while you're actually urinating. Stop the flow once you start it. Stop the flow three times, gradually increasing to five or six each time you urinate.
3. Practice as suggested above. Then try tightening your pelvic floor muscles during intercourse. Your husband will notice the increasing strength of these muscles as you continue to exercise and build them.

4. Practice your Kegel exercises whenever you can—when you're waiting in line, watching TV, doing the dishes, every time you stop at a red light, while you brush your teeth, during other regular everyday activities. Making this a daily habit will help you keep your pelvic floor muscles strong for the rest of your life.

## "I CAN'T GET MY RINGS ON"— EDEMA OR FLUID RETENTION

One of the beautiful benefits of pregnancy you may notice is that your face has a lovely, rosy glow and smooth, wrinkle-free skin. A mild case of edema or fluid rentention—common in pregnancy—is responsible. With the glow, however, you may also get swelling in your ankles, feet, hands, or face. Your rings or shoes may be tight, or you'll feel your eyes have disappeared under their puffy lids. This swelling means you are collecting fluids in your tissues and body cavities.

All women retain fluids during pregnancy, probably due to high levels of water-binding estrogen. If you have ever taken oral contraceptives you may have noticed the same effects. Some fluids go into the blood, causing an increase in blood pressure. As the pregnancy progresses, the pressure on the lower part of the body forces fluid from the veins into the tissue spaces. Unless you're exercising or lying down, the fluid is trapped, resulting in the swelling of the ankles or other extremities that is characteristic of late pregnancy. If the weather is warm, or if you have to stand around on your feet without much other exercise, you may swell more than usual.

Mild edema isn't dangerous. In fact, some studies show that women with uncomplicated edema have larger babies and fewer premature births. But it can be uncomfortable and make you look less than your best. Here are a few suggestions (make sure you get your doctor's approval before following them):

- Make sure your diet doesn't include excessive carbohydrates. Carbohydrates tend to add weight and cause the body to hold water.
- You may need a certain amount of salt during pregnancy so, don't take diuretics or reduce your intake of salt without your doctor's

advice. If your doctor does recommend restricting sodium, make sure you're not taking it in the form of sodium bicarbonate or other medication for indigestion.

- Throughout the day, take rest periods in which you lie down with your feet raised. This reduces pressure and allows the blood and fluid to move back to the heart. Do this as often as possible.
- For puffy eyes, try sleeping with your head elevated on one or two pillows. Or use a remedy that works for a friend of ours: soak tea bags in ice water and gently squeeze out excess liquid; then lie down, close your eyes, and place the bags on your eyes for five minutes.
- Exercise helps to squeeze water from tissue spaces in your blood vessels. It also helps pump blood out of the veins if you have vascular edema. A note of caution here: exercise could be dangerous if you have the kind of severe edema associated with heart failure. So check with your doctor.

| TOXEMIA OR PREECLAMPSIA | MEDICAL ALERT |
|---|---|

While most edema results from normal fluid retention, occasionally it can be the warning sign of toxemia or preeclampsia, a medical condition that can lead to eclampsia, a life-threatening disorder marked by convulsions. Eclampsia has become a rare condition now that more women are getting proper prenatal care, but some women, especially first-time mothers or those who have a poor diet, get mild toxemia under faithful medical supervision. Sometimes it results from the complication of preexisting conditions, such as hypertension in older mothers who have had many births.

The danger signals for toxemia are: excessive or sudden weight gain; marked swelling or fluid rention; severe or continuous headaches; blurred vision; nausea; pain in the abdomen. If you are experiencing any of these symptoms, call your doctor immediately. She will test for a rise in blood pressure or for protein in the urine, and will take the steps necessary to treat the disease before it becomes serious. The treatment might include bed rest, diuretics, and a low-sodium or totally salt-restricted diet. Your doctor's orders should be carefully followed if you have this dangerous disease.

## EXERCISING FOR TWO

Exercise is so helpful in relieving or preventing the problems your pregnant body encounters that we're devoting a whole section to it in this chapter. Because the idea of exercising during pregnancy is still relatively new, you might ask a number of questions: What's the best exercise for me during my pregnancy? Can I start a new sport after I become pregnant? Will any particular exercise hurt me or the baby? Will exercise make childbirth easier for me?

Your obstetrician's approval is the first prerequisite. That should depend on your own medical condition and history. If your pregnancy is complicated, she may ask you to avoid exercises altogether. Even in case of perfectly normal pregnancies with no complications, one doctor's opinion on exercise may differ completely from another's.

Some doctors discourage any sport that jolts the body, especially in the first trimester when the danger of miscarriage is the greatest. Other doctors allow any reasonable exercise throughout the nine months. Very risky sports such as sky-diving, skin-diving (during which the fetus might be deprived of oxygen), hang-gliding, skateboarding, etc. are obviously not in the cards for a pregnant woman. Some doctors give the okay to *starting* certain new sports after you become pregnant, while many doctors believe that beginning a strenuous new sport puts too much strain on a pregnant woman's body and the chance of an accident while engaged in a new sport or exercise is too great.

When you talk to your obstetrician, explain exactly what sport or exercise you'll be doing. If your doctor is a runner or a tennis player, chances are that jogging and tennis will be approved providing your pregnancy is uncomplicated. Most obstetricians encourage women to participate in physical activities during pregnancy since medical research has continually shown that good physical condition results in fewer birth complications. If you are happy with your doctor, follow his advice on your exercise program even when you read arguments on the other side of the question.

What is the overall favorite sport doctors recommend for pregnant women? Swimming, since it exercises all parts of the body while putting no parts under extra strain. You are also very buoyant during pregnancy which makes swimming easier and more fun. Swimming also gets the heart going to supply increased oxygen to your entire body. Try adapting your floor exercises (pp. 132–43) to water. The water resists your movements and makes these exercises more effective.

Because jogging is the fastest growing sport, new studies have been conducted on the pregnant jogger. The results show that strenuous exercise *is* safe for the healthy pregnant woman. You will, however, have to run more slowly than formerly and long-distance or marathon running should be carefully discussed with your obstetrician. Pregnancy seems to slow you down naturally. Liz, the beautiful six-and-a-half-month pregnant runner at the beginning of this chapter remarked, "I was surprised to see that my former eight-minute mile had now become a twelve-minute one!"

Many women worry about the jarring movement of jogging. The fetus, however, is well protected by amniotic fluid, cushioning it against physical shock. A pair of well-padded running shoes will help absorb some of the shock. A supportive bra is also a must for any kind of exercise while you are pregnant.

The vigorous nature of jogging makes some women suspect that it might deprive the fetus of oxygen, blood, or nutrients. This is no cause for concern: evidence shows that during brisk exercise the baby will receive no less than what it needs. Blood flow is preferentially increased to the pregnant uterus before it passes to most of the other organs.

Be smart about your limits in any sport or exercise. If you experience any pain, nausea, dizziness, or spotting, stop immediately and rest in bed until you can reach your doctor. Let your body be a guide. If you are exercising at a health club, don't use a sauna. Studies show that overheating during the first months of pregnancy can cause birth defects.

You will have to eat more than the nonathletic woman. While the moderately active average pregnant woman requires 2,300 calories, if you are doing strenuous exercise you will have to add, say, 100 calories for each mile you run. Just fifteen minutes of backstrokes uses up 140 calories and one hour of walking uses up 270 calories.

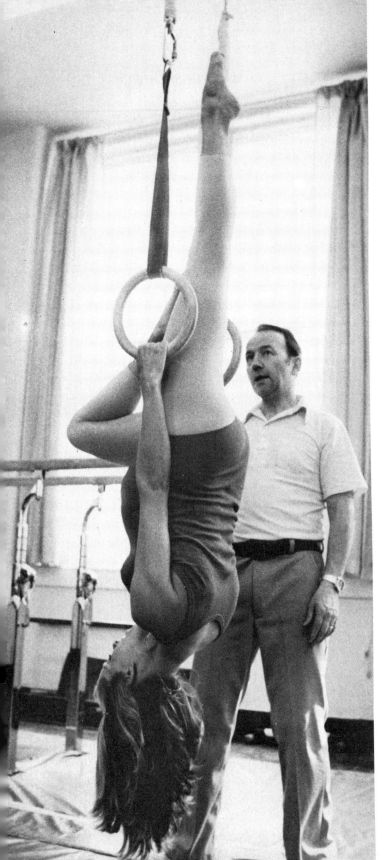

Here's Joanne viewing the world with a new perspective at a special prenatal class with her instructor, Werner. She's eight months pregnant and perfectly fit to hang upside-down on the rings since she was doing this exercise for years before she became pregnant with her second child.

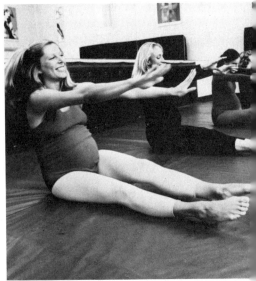

Joanne does a "fanny walk" to firm up hip, thighs, and fanny.

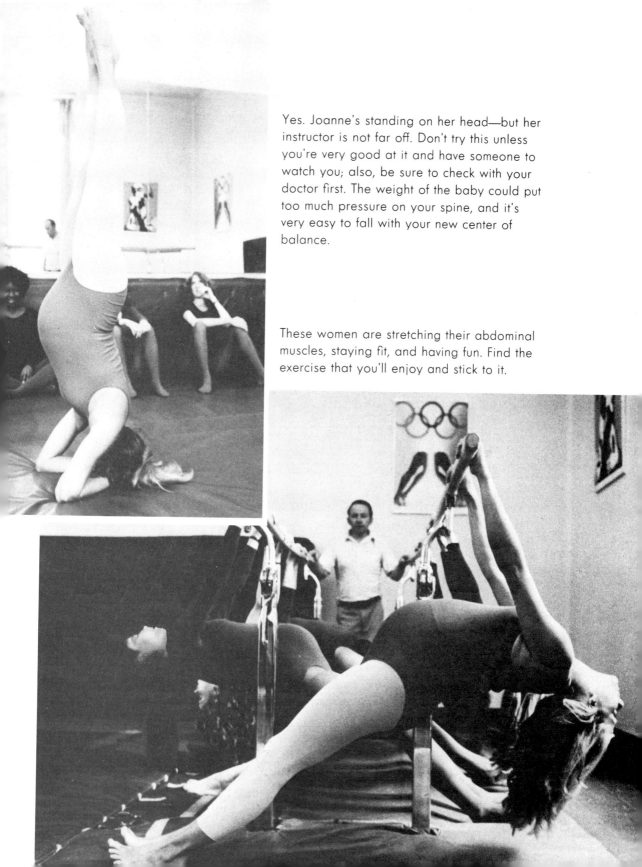

Yes. Joanne's standing on her head—but her instructor is not far off. Don't try this unless you're very good at it and have someone to watch you; also, be sure to check with your doctor first. The weight of the baby could put too much pressure on your spine, and it's very easy to fall with your new center of balance.

These women are stretching their abdominal muscles, staying fit, and having fun. Find the exercise that you'll enjoy and stick to it.

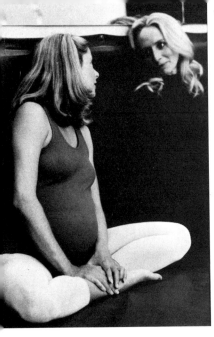

The tailor position is very natural and comfortable for relaxing and talking with other pregnant women in the class. It also stretches the inner thigh muscles, which aid during childbirth.

Joanne's instructor lifts her legs and pelvis to relieve pressure on the pelvic floor and venous vein. Ask your husband to do this for you.

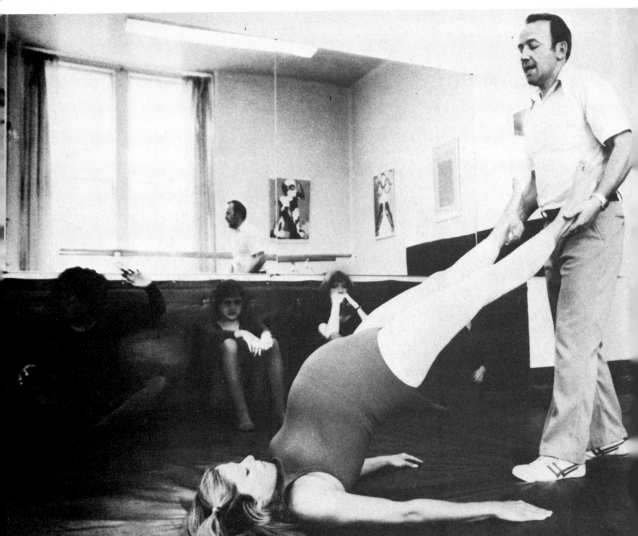

WARM-UP FOR EXERCISE. As we have mentioned, certain hormones of pregnancy—especially a well-named one called relaxin—cause your joint tissues to relax and become looser. The purpose of this, it is believed, is to relax the pelvic joint tissue to prepare the body for delivery. These hormones succeed in slightly loosening all the connective tissues throughout the body. This puts your body at a disadvantage. If your joints are looser, they're also weaker.

This has to be kept in mind when you exercise. A warm-up before exercising is especially important so that the joints become lubricated and that their collagen tissues contract, increasing their strength. You may tire more easily and find that your exercise rate slows down as your due date approaches. Take clues from your body and do as it says.

PRENATAL EXERCISE CLASS. One of the best recommendations we can give you is to take a prenatal exercise class. (These are not to be confused with prepared-childbirth classes, although we highly recommend these classes as well for an easier, more enjoyable, and educated birth experience.) You can start prenatal exercises when you first learn you are pregnant. Prenatal exercise classes teach you how to move while you are pregnant as well as helping you to strengthen and limber up your changing body. You'll have a wonderful time talking to other expectant mothers, comparing tummies, exchanging complaints and joys, and learning from others' experiences. Along with exercise, a group therapy will emerge and you will stop feeling you are the only pregnant woman in the world. And an exercise class is a chance to do something just for yourself plus make yourself fit and pretty at the same time.

If you don't know of a prenatal exercise class check with your prepared-childbirth instructor, your community center, or your hospital. Many YWCAs are now offering prenatal exercise courses.

Beyond making friends, why is exercise during pregnancy so important? Here are a few reasons:

- Exercise *prepares* your body for the physical stress of pregnancy. Although pregnancy is a natural condition, it does tax the body muscles, ligaments, tissues, etc., especially in the back, pelvic area, legs, feet, and hips. Exercise is a buffer for these new stresses on the body.

- Exercise helps *prevent* problems associated with pregnancy, such as a relaxed pelvic area, chronic back problems, poor urine control, and other large and little annoyances. Heredity and other factors also play roles, but exercise can often be the decisive preventative for those problems.

- Exercise *energizes* you so that you don't tire so easily during pregnancy. This vigor extends to other parts of life such as lovemaking and being an energetic and cheerful mother for your other children. Exercise also makes you feel good!

- Whether exercise *helps you in labor and delivery* is a debated point. Some experts believe the uterus does all the work and your muscle tone doesn't affect your delivery. If you don't exercise at all you will still be able to have a perfectly normal delivery. On the other hand, exercise does strengthen your entire body. Women who exercise will not be making the first demands on their bodies during labor. They have worked their bodies before and are confident they can perform. If there is a lot of pushing involved in your delivery, you will certainly benefit from strong abdominal muscles.

- Exercise *relaxes* you by providing an outlet for emotional and physical tensions.

- Proper exercises *teach you how to breathe* to maximize the use of oxygen. This will make the prepared-childbirth techniques easier to master. The growing baby benefits as well.

- Exercise teaches *grace and good posture*—essentials for beauty and health.

- A physically fit body—especially during pregnancy—is *sexy*. Staying well-toned, strong, and active is all part of the changing image of pregnant women. Exercising, by increasing blood circulation, gives your skin a pretty glow all over. A pregnant woman who is also fit and healthy is glamorous!

- "The real reward," said Lorence, the physical fitness expert of Gala Fitness Studios in New York City, "is after the baby's born. Women who have been exercising during pregnancy get *back into shape* much more easily than those who don't. I love seeing these women coming in three weeks after the birth of their baby and looking beautiful, slim, and fit again!"

NO-NO EXERCISES. There are certain exercises you *shouldn't* do while you're pregnant. They can put strain on areas of your body which are already under too much stress. The softened ligaments and tissues due to pregnancy hormones we mentioned earlier contribute to the weakening of these areas.

1. Don't do leg raises from a prone position. The strain on your spinal joints is too great.
2. Don't do deep knee bends. Your knees are a very delicate part of your body and are under extra strain during pregnancy.
(Many exercise experts warn against knee bends at any time.)
3. Don't do the "rocking horse" (lying on your stomach, reaching back to your ankles, and then rocking back and forth). Any exercise that hollows the back is terrible for the pregnant woman. The abdominal muscles as well as the back muscles are strained in this exercise.
4. Don't do sit-ups with outstretched legs. They too overstrain the back muscles. Sit-ups before or after pregnancy should always be done with knees bent.
5. Most pregnant women find that exercising on their stomachs becomes extremely uncomfortable once they begin to show. Exercises that require you to get up on your shoulders should also be avoided unless you are used to them. Your weight is too unwieldy as pregnancy progresses and you may fall.

## YOUR BEAUTIFUL PREGNANT BODY

At the end of nine months you look at your body in the mirror in utter amazement. It's fascinating. Its fecundity and overripeness are poetic, its sheer bulk and size almost silly. You're beautiful—but the beauty of your well-exercised body goes beyond rosy glow, pretty nails, and full glorious breasts. Your body's blueprint and the endocrinological changes of adolescence and menstruation have led you up to this one reproductive event.

The best advice on how to handle the body changes, aches, and pains of pregnancy is: Be philosophical. Be educated and practice preventive medicine. If you have a problem tend to it promptly. And don't dwell on it. Any discomforts you may have suffered now become secondary to the promise of new life.

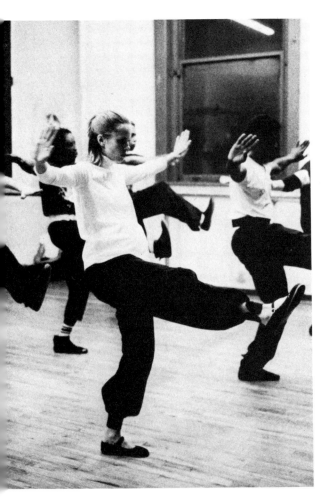

Lynne attends a class in T'ai Chi Ch'uan, a centuries-old martial art teaching combat training but designed to be a meditative yoga form as well. It stresses passivity to overcome aggression. This class provides the stretching exercises of yoga and helps strengthen legs and arms—all beneficial for pregnancy. The class is held right next door to Lynne's apartment. Choose an exercise class that's close and convenient for you.

## PRENATAL EXERCISES

The following exercises were created as a special program for us by Diana Simkin, a young woman who has conducted pre- and postnatal exercise classes in New York City since 1974. Diana Simkin has a master's degree in dance education from New York University and is a Lamaze instructor. She is a protégé of Elisabeth Bing, the noted prepared-childbirth expert and author.

All the following exercises can be done throughout your pregnancy. Remember to check with your doctor before starting any exercise program. Stop exercising if you experience pain or spotting at any point. Tell your obstetrician about this pain and find out which exercises you can safely continue.

Try to keep a steady breathing pattern throughout each exercise, unless the exercise has special breathing instructions. Never hold your breath while exercising—it will only increase tension and make exercising more difficult.

Make these exercises a daily ritual during your nine months. Some women find they adhere to their exercise schedule if they have a special time and place, such as during the six o'clock news or as soon as they get up in the morning. Other women, who find themselves resistant to schedules and must-dos, find they do these exercises, despite themselves, by varying the time and place of exercises. Try them one day in front of the TV, the next day in the quiet of the bedroom, or even in the kitchen to a radio while the stew is simmering. Try to squeeze in a session every day. Almost all the women we talked to felt that putting on a leotard was the single most important step in getting started! Exercise will make your body feel good and your glow even rosier. Have fun.

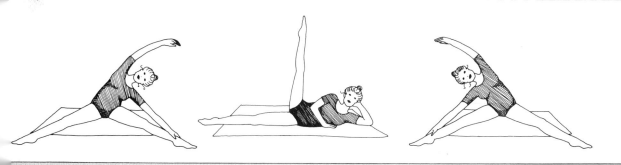

## 1. PELVIC TILT

**Purpose: to strengthen the abdomen and pelvic floor, and to lengthen and relax the lower back muscles.**

Lie on your back with your knees bent and feet placed about six inches apart. Place your hands on your abdomen. Take a slow, deep breath in and feel your abdomen expand beneath your fingers. Then breathe out, flattening and tightening your abdomen at the same time, as if you were pushing the air out of the abdomen. Repeat this 5 times.

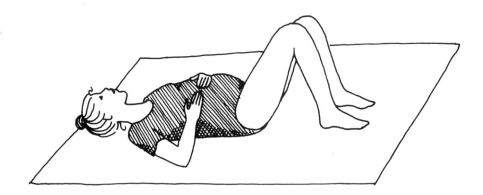

In the same position, take a deep breath in. As you exhale this time, pull in the abdomen as before, tighten the pelvic floor (all the muscles around the vagina), and lightly tighten the buttocks and the backs of the thighs. (You'll feel your lower back flatten against the floor.) Then inhale, gently relaxing all the muscles. Repeat this 8 times.

## 2. LEG STRETCHES

**Purpose: to stretch and strengthen the muscles in the legs, feet, and abdomen.**

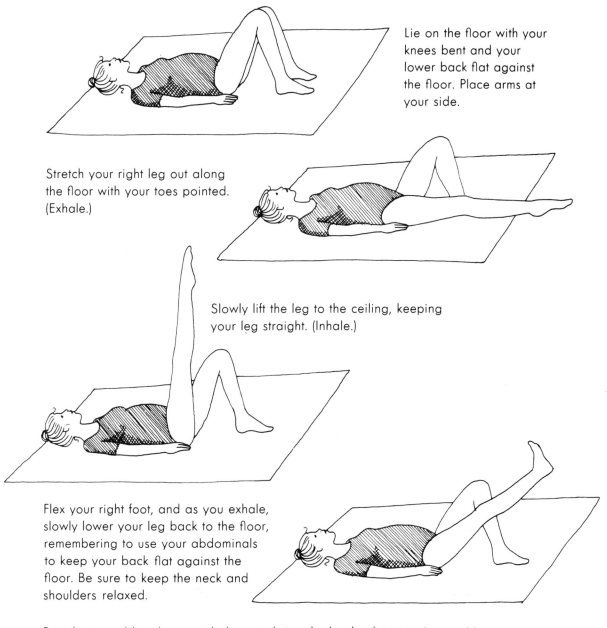

Lie on the floor with your knees bent and your lower back flat against the floor. Place arms at your side.

Stretch your right leg out along the floor with your toes pointed. (Exhale.)

Slowly lift the leg to the ceiling, keeping your leg straight. (Inhale.)

Flex your right foot, and as you exhale, slowly lower your leg back to the floor, remembering to use your abdominals to keep your back flat against the floor. Be sure to keep the neck and shoulders relaxed.

Breathe in and bend your right knee to bring the leg back to starting position. Change legs and repeat exercise with left leg. Repeat this 5 times for each leg.

## 3. SIDE KNEE ROLLS

**Purpose: to increase tone and flexibility in the waist and hips.**

Lie on your back with your knees bent, your lower back flat against the floor. Place your arms out to the sides at shoulder height, with palms facing down to the floor.

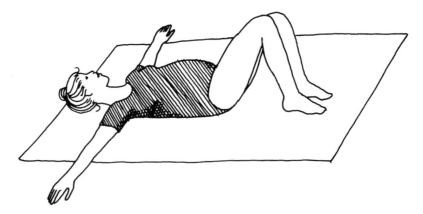

Keeping your feet on the floor and your arms in place, roll your knees from side to side in one slow continuous motion. Breathe in as your knees descend to the floor and breathe out as you bring them up, using your abdominal muscles to roll your back flat to the floor each time. Keep neck and shoulders relaxed. Repeat this 10 times—5 times on each side.

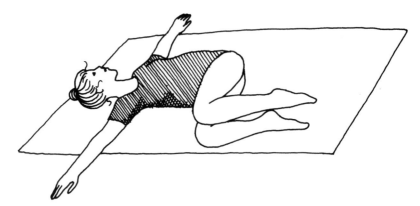

## 4. THE V STRETCH

**Purpose:** to strengthen the abdomen, thighs, and feet.
**NOTE:** especially helpful for stretching and strengthening inner thigh muscles used during delivery.

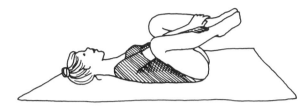

Lie down with your lower back flat against the floor. Bend your knees and hold your ankles with your hands inside your legs. Take a deep breath.

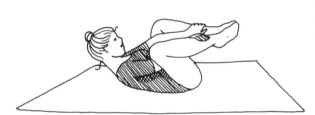

Exhaling, lift your head and upper back up off the floor, and pull your chin in to your chest. Make sure to keep your abdomen flat—don't let it bulge. At the same time, press thighs open with your elbows. Hold a couple of seconds. Release your head and shoulders back down to the floor and return to the first position.

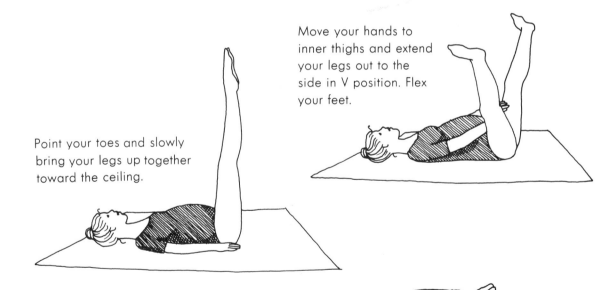

Move your hands to inner thighs and extend your legs out to the side in V position. Flex your feet.

Point your toes and slowly bring your legs up together toward the ceiling.

Gently bend your knees and hold your ankles to return to the first position. Repeat this 5 times.

## 5. PELVIC ROLL

**Purpose:** to work the same areas as the Pelvic Tilt in addition to increasing flexibility of the back area.
**NOTE:** this exercise will help relieve backaches.

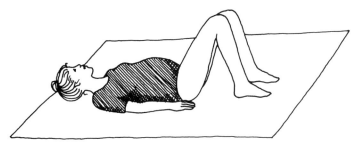

Lie flat on the floor with your knees bent and feet placed six inches apart. Place arms by your side.

Slowly peel your back off the floor, starting with the buttocks, then the waist, middle back, and finally the upper back. If this is done correctly, there should be a straight line from your shoulders to your knees.

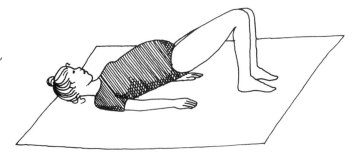

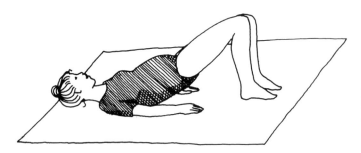

Next, slowly roll your back down to the floor, starting with your upper back and ribs, then the middle back, waist, and finally the buttocks. Remember to keep breathing regularly throughout this exercise. Repeat this 6 times.

## 6. SIDE LEG STRETCHES

**Purpose: to firm the inner thighs.**

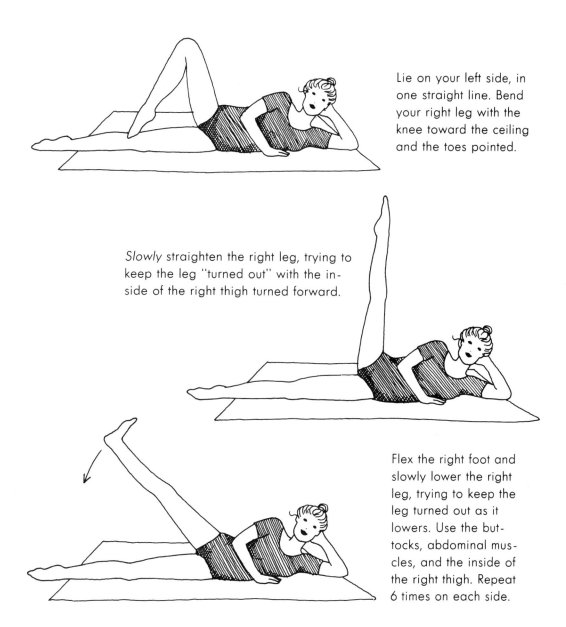

Lie on your left side, in one straight line. Bend your right leg with the knee toward the ceiling and the toes pointed.

*Slowly* straighten the right leg, trying to keep the leg "turned out" with the inside of the right thigh turned forward.

Flex the right foot and slowly lower the right leg, trying to keep the leg turned out as it lowers. Use the buttocks, abdominal muscles, and the inside of the right thigh. Repeat 6 times on each side.

## 7. BODY CIRCLES

**Purpose: to relax the neck, shoulder, and back, and to tone the ribs and waistline.**

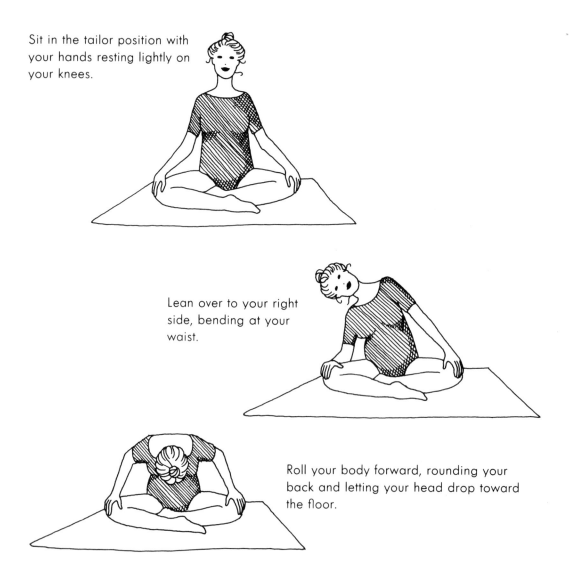

Sit in the tailor position with your hands resting lightly on your knees.

Lean over to your right side, bending at your waist.

Roll your body forward, rounding your back and letting your head drop toward the floor.

Roll your body to the left side, and then back up to the center position in which you started. Repeat this 6 times, alternating direction.

## 8. FLEXING AND POINTING

**Purpose: to strengthen the feet, arches, ankles, and calves.**
**NOTE: this exercise is good if you suffer from leg cramps.**

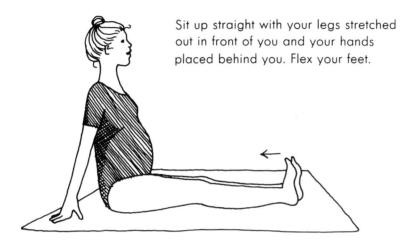

Sit up straight with your legs stretched out in front of you and your hands placed behind you. Flex your feet.

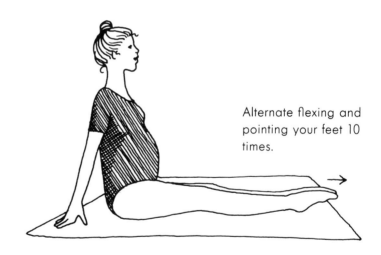

Alternate flexing and pointing your feet 10 times.

## 9. SIDE STRETCHES

**Purpose: to tone and stretch the torso, waist, and thighs.**

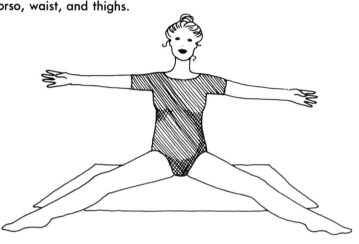

Sit tall with your legs and arms out to the sides. Remember, only take the legs to where *you* can sit *comfortably*. It's not important to open the legs very wide.

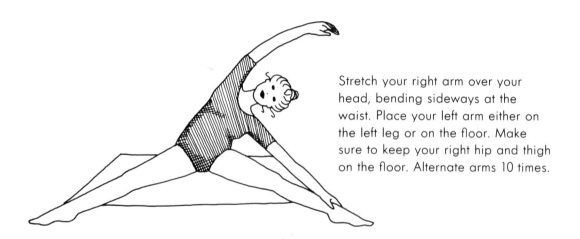

Stretch your right arm over your head, bending sideways at the waist. Place your left arm either on the left leg or on the floor. Make sure to keep your right hip and thigh on the floor. Alternate arms 10 times.

Come back to center, using your abdomen to bring you up and to help support your back. Then lean your head, arms, and back forward and relax in that position for about two to three minutes. Roll up to center position as shown in the first illustration.

## 10. BREAST EXERCISE

Purpose: to strengthen the pectoral muscles and help strengthen upper arm and back muscles.
NOTE: this is also a good exercise to do postpartum.

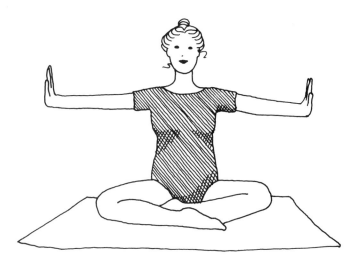

Sit in the tailor position and place your arms out to the side just below shoulder height. Flex your hands and push out as if you were pressing against an imaginary wall.

Make tiny circles with your arms, at the same time moving them slowly toward each other until they are in front of you. Then reverse the circles and open the arms again out to the sides. Make sure to keep your back straight and your body still. Move your arms from your back, not your shoulders, which stay relaxed. Repeat 4 times.

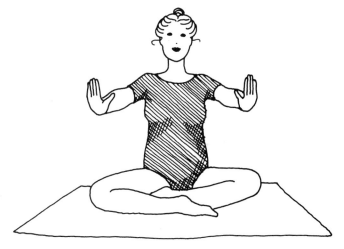

## 11. HEAD AND SHOULDER ROLLS

**Purpose:** to relieve tension in the neck and shoulders.

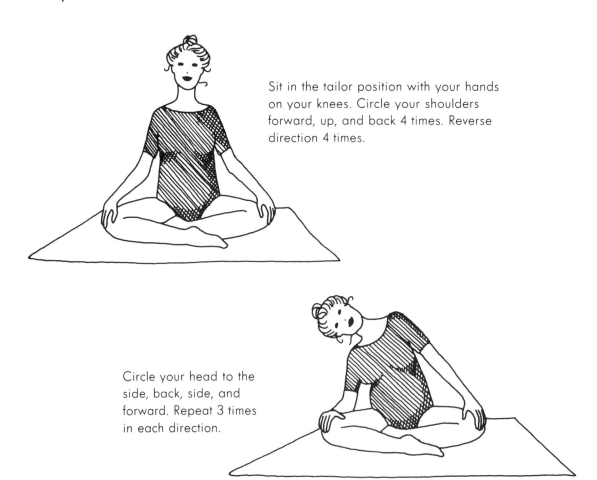

Sit in the tailor position with your hands on your knees. Circle your shoulders forward, up, and back 4 times. Reverse direction 4 times.

Circle your head to the side, back, side, and forward. Repeat 3 times in each direction.

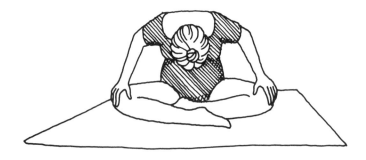

## 12. RELAXATION EXERCISE

**Purpose:** to relax the spine, back, shoulders, and neck.

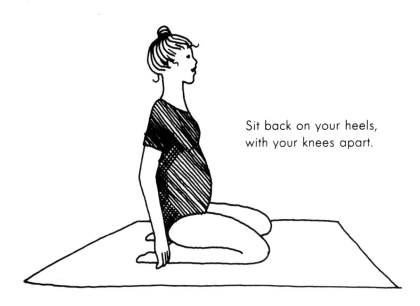

Sit back on your heels, with your knees apart.

Lean forward and let your forehead rest on the floor. Arms can be left at your side or stretched out in front of you. Relax there for a minute or two, breathing slowly and deeply.

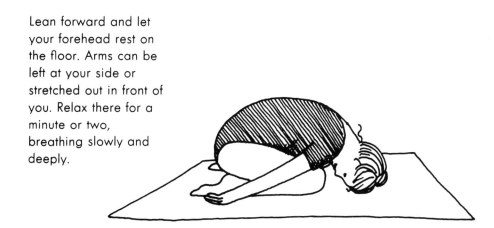

# CHAPTER ·V·

# *Fashion During Pregnancy*

"WHAT I LOVE ABOUT BEING PREGNANT is the total freedom to create any look I like," says Mary Ann, a five-month-pregnant woman from Los Angeles. "It's a kind of reverse psychology. Now that I don't feel compelled to follow the current fashions, I'm actually trying more of them. I've found that pregnancy's been a time to live out fashion fantasies—it's great!"

Isn't it true! Antique clothes, designer clothes, maternity clothes, trendy clothes—any clothes that accommodate your growing tummy prettily—are terrific for making you look and feel sexy and lovely-to-look-at during pregnancy. Pregnancy is a time to show off your good looks, your big stomach, and all the vitality pregnancy has endowed you with. When you stop to think about it, nine months is a short time—so dress yourself up for the occasion. You'll feel and, of course, you'll look better if you use imagination, common sense, wit, and instinct for glamor while outfitting yourself these nine months.

This chapter gives only general guidelines to fashion during pregnancy. Fashions change in the wink of St. Laurent's eye—and although the loose, billowy look of the last few years carried many a mother-to-be all the way through pregnancy, today's silhouette is cut much closer to the body.

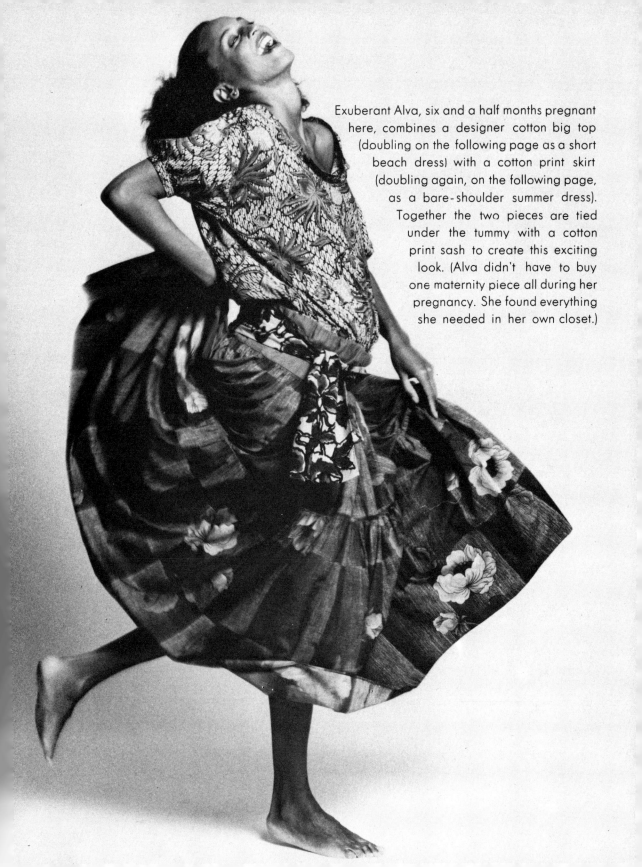

Exuberant Alva, six and a half months pregnant here, combines a designer cotton big top (doubling on the following page as a short beach dress) with a cotton print skirt (doubling again, on the following page, as a bare-shoulder summer dress). Together the two pieces are tied under the tummy with a cotton print sash to create this exciting look. (Alva didn't have to buy one maternity piece all during her pregnancy. She found everything she needed in her own closet.)

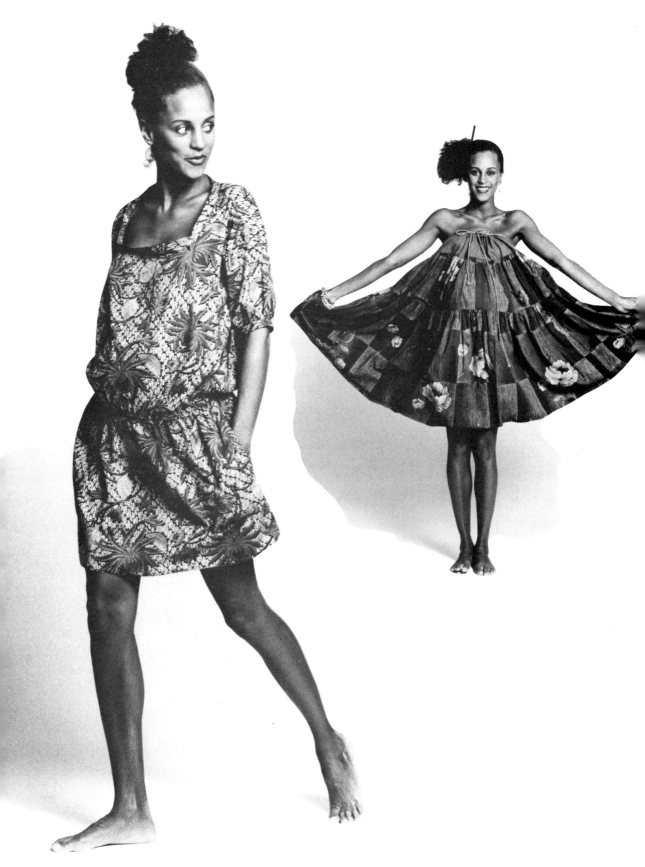

Even so, you can count on certain classic styles that can be adapted for your pregnancy, and you can take advantage of some of the inventive and elegant clothes designed specifically for your pregnant body.

## DO I NEED A WHOLE NEW WARDROBE?

For the nine months of your pregnancy you will need enough clothes to carry you through all your personal, professional, and social obligations feeling as poised and well-dressed as you do when you're not pregnant. That doesn't mean you have to start from scratch: begin with a tough scrutiny of the clothes you already own. Look through all the clothes in your closet and dresser: do you have any full dresses normally worn either with or without a belt? These are often ideal maternity dresses. Do you have any full jumpers or evening caftans which could serve at some point during your pregnancy? What about silk or cotton tunics which you've worn over pants, billowy cotton shirts, or long loose T-shirts? Do you have any "fat clothes"—clothes from a period in which you weighed more? Think about ways to make them all work for you as you read about adapting your wardrobe.

The baby doesn't show immediately, of course, so nature gives you a chance to ease into a fuller look slowly. Although each woman "shows" at a different time and in a different way, generally speaking, you should be able to wear your usual clothes for the first two to four months. (Even those women who gain little weight find their body weight redistributes itself in the first three to four months and their clothes fit poorly.) After the third or fourth month, you'll probably find that even your loosest clothes won't work. Only a few lucky women don't have to buy any maternity clothes, save some new underwear or a pair of maternity blue jeans. Alva, shown at the beginning of this chapter, was one of them—during her pregnancy, clothes were full and Alva's own style tended towards a loose, unstructured look, so it was easy for her to get away with nonmaternity clothes. Most of us will buy some maternity clothes during pregnancy, however. Judy, a thirty-two-year-old, pregnant with her second child, said,

"I bought more maternity clothes this time than the last. I think many women get into a martyr trap like I did the first time. They try to get along on as little as possible. By the seventh or eighth month of my last pregnancy, I was sick to death of the two or three outfits I'd allowed myself and yet felt I'd only get two months' use out of something I'd buy at that point. During my second pregnancy I started buying maternity clothes earlier and have enjoyed them all the way through."

"WHEN WILL I NEED WHAT?"
TWO IMPORTANT GROWTH STAGES

This doesn't mean that you have to wear maternity clothes after your first visit to the doctor. Up to your second to fourth month you will probably be wearing your regular clothes, although your bust and/or tummy will be growing quickly. Once you've started growing out of these clothes, you'll be dressing for two separate stages of growth.

You will have to make the first alterations in your clothing during the middle part of pregnancy—roughly the second trimester. During this period you can still wear some of your skirts unzipped under a loose-fitting top, or expand your pants with an elastic band sewn into the waistband. This, at first, may make you feel strangely exposed, or unfinished, but you soon get used to it. If you have some full dresses you can go right on wearing them for the time being. But you may have to buy some dresses or tops at this stage—or you may want to show off your new pregnant look. Make sure that anything you buy now is big enough for a nine-month-pregnant you. Use the pillow some maternity shops provide to help you judge your full-term size; *no one* believes just how big she is going to be. If you buy maternity clothes that you *do* grow out of, don't despair. They can be used in the first few months postpartum when your body is still involuting (or returning to its original size), while you're nursing or still overweight. Many women are astonished when they can't fit into their size-eight pants right after delivery. They do get back to their original size eventually. (A note on planning: if you're intending to nurse your baby and want to wear your maternity clothes during the first few months postpartum, make sure you have lots of pieces that button down the front or lift up easily from the bottom.)

Around about your sixth month you will enter the stage of full-bloom pregnancy. No one will mistake you for having a weight problem or miss the fact that you are pregnant. This is the point when, if you haven't already done so, you'll probably have to invest in some special clothes to keep you pretty and comfy.

You can find fashionable maternity clothes from many sources today, including maternity shops. Maternity designers no longer expect women to apologize for pregnancy by wearing clothes that hide it. They no longer try to surround women with ruffles, smocking, and ribbons that make them look more like babies than mothers. Maternity clothes designers, and top-name dress and sportswear designers who have recently entered the maternity market, are translating today's fashion into the idiom of maternity clothes. They make glamorous clothes that say you are proud to be pregnant. This doesn't mean you should wrap yourself in revealing jersey, nor does it mean you must make your tummy the overwhelming focus of your look. *You* are still the star.

## WHERE TO FIND MATERNITY CLOTHES

When you've discovered that your regular clothes just won't fit anymore, and you decide to start assembling your new look as mother-to-be, where do you go? By now you know where you like to shop; you've found the fashion boutique or discount house or antique clothes dealer whose style matches yours. But what about maternity clothes?

The best quality maternity clothes are found in the small specialty maternity shops, but the maternity departments of large department stores are also fine. Recently department stores have upgraded their maternity depart-

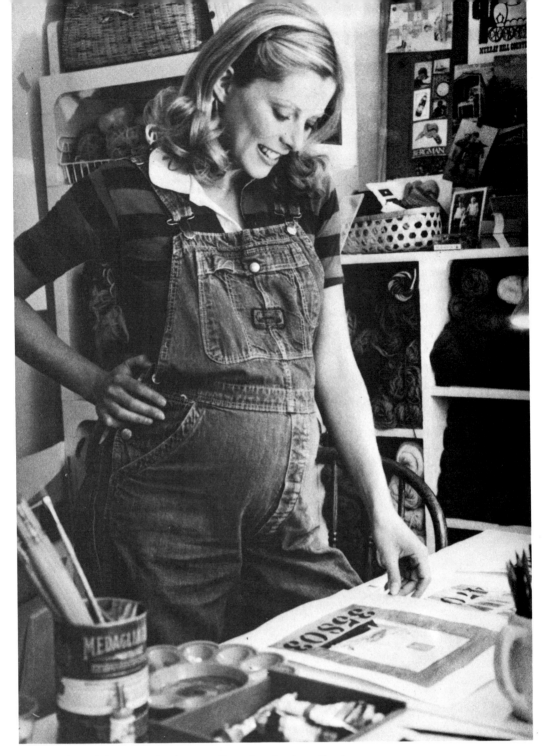
Joanne found these worker's overalls in her husband's closet.

ments to include better quality clothes made of finer fabrics with more detail work.

Where else can you go for maternity clothes? Try these:

- Your husband's closet is one of the best sources for loose-fitting shirts, jackets, even pants (see Joanne, *opposite,* in her husband's overalls).
- Your sewing machine. If you sew, make your own maternity clothes in the fabrics you like best. Use maternity or regular big look patterns.
- Friends. They love to get rid of their old maternity clothes and like to know they're going for a good cause.
- Five-and-ten-cent stores—more bargains! Get your cotton underwear here too.
- Thrift shops—bargains galore.
- Attics. What Mom didn't have, your grandma may have.
- Regular dress departments for full-look dresses.
- Half-size department in large stores.
- Lingerie departments that carry lots of loose-fitting clothes.
- Stores or boutiques specializing in various ethnic looks such as caftans, Greek cotton shirts, drawstring pants, African dashikis, Moroccan cotton djellabas, Japanese kimonos, and full tunic tops with mandarin collars.


## ASSEMBLING YOUR NEW WARDROBE

What new maternity items you need depends on your life-style: whether you're working or not; whether you live in a city, suburbs, or country; how limited your budget is; through how many seasons you'll be pregnant. For the last topic, our advice is to buy for one season only—winter or summer—and try to make those clothes do for the in-between months. If your budget is limited, buy less and borrow more, start sewing, or bargain-hunting in the places mentioned in the previous section. For city life, obviously, you'll need more dressy clothes and for country life, the emphasis is on casual. We have two lists of wardrobe basics; one for the working woman, and one for the woman who stays at home. Consult these for ideas as to what you will need.

## BASIC WARDROBE CHECKLIST FOR WORKING WOMEN

At no time in your working life is it more important to look well-dressed and attractive than during your pregnancy. Whether you plan to stop working indefinitely when the baby comes or you expect to return to work six weeks after the baby's birth, the image you project during your pregnancy should be as poised and professional as ever. There are plenty of people—coworkers and competitors—who will imagine you've dropped out of competition by "fulfilling your biological destiny." You don't want to give them any ammunition.

Invest in a wardrobe that says what you already know: that you can be a mother and an efficient and effective worker at the same time. Because you'll be filling more roles, you'll need clothes that work more ways. Choose quality clothes whenever possible. You'll find they wear better and will hold their shape during the long months. Many women prefer lighter fabrics because they relieve the warmth of pregnancy. Wash-and-wear fabrics can be lifesavers for a busy working woman. This is the basic wardrobe checklist for the working woman:

- ☐ 3 maternity dresses or full-look dresses which can be used for pregnancy
- ☐ 2 jumpers
- ☐ 1 coordinated pants outfit such as a blazer or top and pants in a good fabric
- ☐ 1 more pair of slacks
- ☐ 3–4 tops that will work with slacks or long cotton T-shirts for casual wear
- ☐ 1 pair of maternity jeans
- ☐ 1 at-home caftan
- ☐ 1 cocktail dress or evening gown

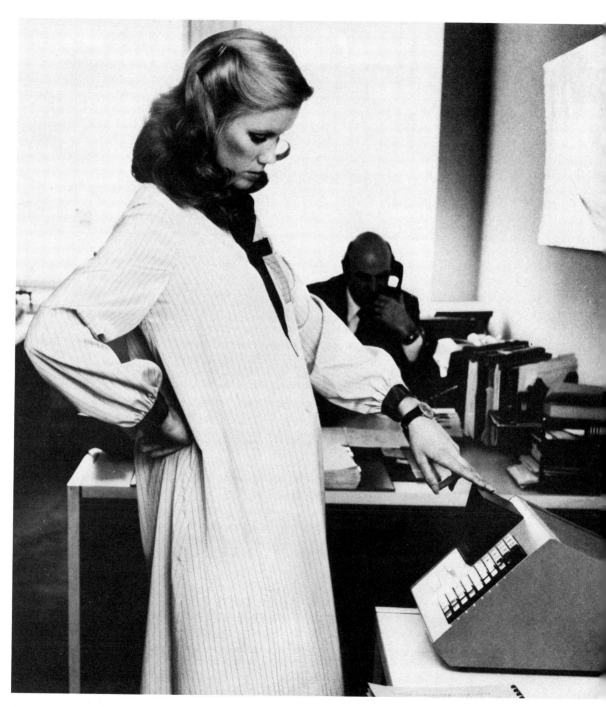

Office wear: Liz, six months pregnant here, chooses the conservative pin-
stripe look—a brown and cream silky dress that's as soft and feminine as
can be. The stripes are perfect to slim down the bulky look of a woman in
her last months of pregnancy.

☐ 2 maternity slips (full or half)
☐ 3 bras
☐ 6 pairs, at least, of maternity or queen-sized pantyhose

## BASIC WARDROBE CHECKLIST FOR
## THE NONWORKING WOMAN

If you aren't working, you have more flexibility about what you choose to wear. If you are active in the community and must attend meetings or go out a lot in the evening you need more than what is included here. If life revolves around your home and you don't go out much, you'll need less. Wash-and-wear fabrics and no-iron fabrics save on cleaning costs and time. Choose fabrics that will hold their shape after many months of wear. Here are the absolute basics:

☐ 1 daytime dress
☐ 1 jumper
☐ 2 pairs maternity slacks
☐ 4–5 maternity tops
☐ 1 pair maternity jeans
☐ 1 at-home caftan
☐ 1 cocktail dress or evening gown
☐ 1 maternity slip
☐ 3 bras
☐ 4 pairs of maternity or queen-sized pantyhose

## DRESSES

Dresses, as you'll eventually find out, are the basic pieces of maternity wear. Whether for work or other daytime or evening wear, they are the comfortable and practical solution for pregnant dressing: they make you look

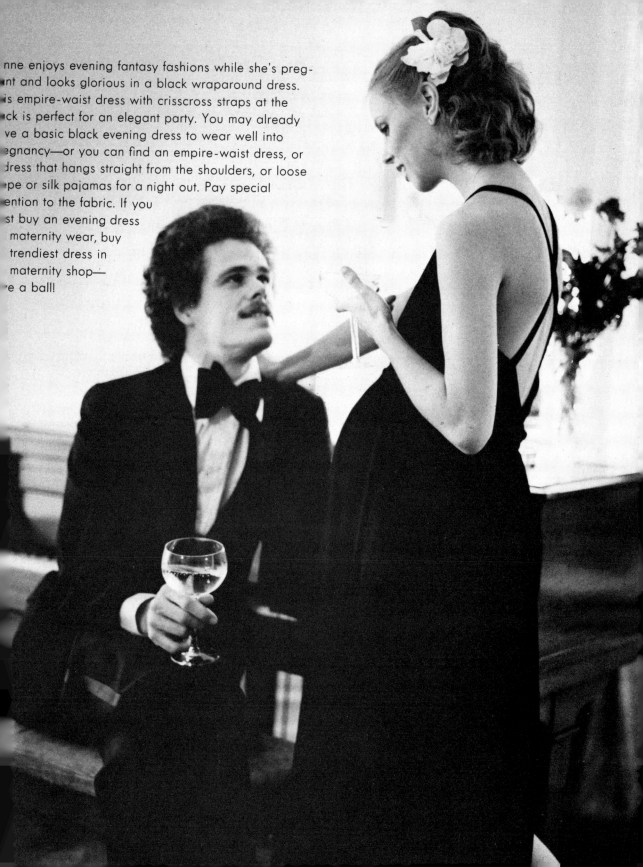

nne enjoys evening fantasy fashions while she's preg-
nt and looks glorious in a black wraparound dress.
is empire-waist dress with crisscross straps at the
ck is perfect for an elegant party. You may already
ve a basic black evening dress to wear well into
egnancy—or you can find an empire-waist dress, or
dress that hangs straight from the shoulders, or loose
pe or silk pajamas for a night out. Pay special
ention to the fabric. If you
st buy an evening dress
maternity wear, buy
trendiest dress in
maternity shop—
e a ball!

pulled-together, unfussy, and elegant. A maternity buyer for a large department store gave us these tips:

- One of the best dress silhouettes you can choose is the classic full A-line that drops from the shoulder and falls gently over your body. It flatters your form rather than making it look bulbous. A full smock look is also pretty for pregnancy.
- The loose empire look works well in dresses, but avoid dresses that tie tightly under the bust, emphasizing both large breasts and big abdomen (the "sack-of-potatoes" look).
- Make sure the dress bust size is large enough to accommodate your growing breasts, which often get fuller until the sixth month. In fact, avoid snug-fitting bodices whenever possible. Besides making you look lumpy, tightness around the bust can chafe and (according to dermatologists) cause skin problems around the breasts. But don't buy your dresses two sizes too big: the fit of the shoulders and armhole area won't change throughout your pregnancy.
- Don't buy a dress with a waistline, even if it is large enough to fit. It will look silly. If you buy a full dress with an optional belt to double as a maternity dress, make sure it looks well unbelted and has enough room for your growing baby.
- If you are wearing—or buying—nonmaternity dresses, remember that, depending on how closely they are cut, they will tend to hike up in the front at a certain point in your pregnancy. The front hem lines of most maternity dresses dip one to one and a half inches, depending on the fullness of the skirt. The fuller the dress, the less dip necessary. You might think about letting down the front hemlines of any dress for which this would be a problem.
- Jumpers are one of the best investments you can make. You can dress a jumper up with a silk shirt (unbuttoned underneath over the stomach) or dress it down with a turtleneck.
- Stand straight in your clothes. This makes you look wonderful no matter what you wear.
- Here's an extravagant pick-me-up: Splurge on a pretty new dress for the last month or two of pregnancy.

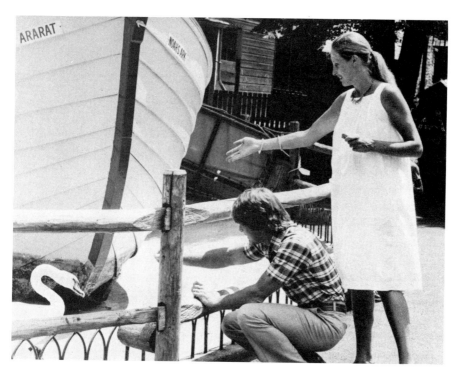

Almost everyone has a loose-fitting jumper or sundress in her closet that can easily be converted for maternity wear.

## TOPS

You probably have more tops that can be converted to maternity-wear than any other item. Check your closet right now to see what you can use. Rule number one for tops or blouses is: make sure the top covers your entire abdomen and doesn't pull up in the front. It's even better to wear a shirt that falls below the crotch area, since shorter tops draw the eye to the crotch or to the behind. (Thank heaven designers are now making maternity tops that also cover the fanny.) Rules number two and three are the same ones that apply to dresses: don't buy tops too big in the armhole and shoulder area, and keep the line simple. After that, let your taste and imagination decide. Many ethnic shirts are perfect for pregnancy because of their full cut. Or you may want to buy some soft, silky maternity blouses that flatter you and add versatility to your wardrobe.

Judy Loeb, a successful designer and the originator of Sweet Mama maternity clothes, suggests that for a pulled-together look, tops and pants and tops and skirts should be matched. The total look is neater (you're one color, or at least two coordinating colors, from top to bottom) and smarter for the working woman.

PANTS

During the first trimester and perhaps into the beginning of the second trimester, you can probably wear your usual pants. When you are no longer able to zip your pants all the way up, open the zipper and sew a piece of one-and-a-half inch elastic to either side of the waistband to hold up your open pants. Or replace the zipper with a V-shaped elastic panel made especially for maternity pants and found at most sewing stores. If you have a pair of pants with an elastic waistband, you may be able to wear them longer—until the waist becomes too binding. You can then sew in a longer piece of elastic to make the waist looser.

When the time comes to buy maternity pants, you have two basic types to choose from. Traditionally styled maternity pants have a loose elastic waistband with a stretch panel across the front. These pants are usually suitable all the way through pregnancy. The newer fly-front maternity pants have a zipper, an elastic waist band, and a V-shaped stretch panel on each side. These pants fit more snugly than the traditional style and are good only until the fifth or sixth month.

Whichever you prefer, don't buy maternity pants with a very wide elastic waistband—most women find these uncomfortably binding. And remember that you may have to take the next size in maternity slacks if you have gained weight in your thighs and fanny.

If you are discouraged by the available selection of maternity pants, take your favorite pair of pants to a good seamstress to have them copied in maternity slacks. Choose a good gabardine or another fine fabric that you

*Opposite page:* Alva looks great wearing a silk man-tailored shirt, a man's vest and handkerchief from the thrift shop, and a pair of designer jersey pants with an elastic expandable waist. The bag is from one of her modeling trips to Senegal. Her shoes are loafers. Alva finds their low heels comfortable.

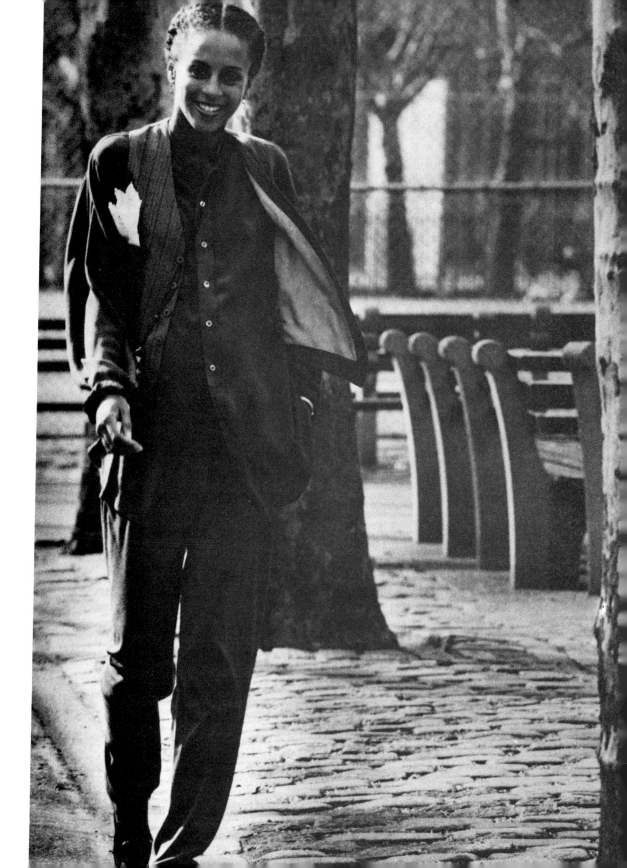

wouldn't find in ready-to-wear maternity slacks. These pants are terrific for the working woman who must look her best every day. For more casual wear, you might try a pair of nonmaternity drawstring pants. They're often prettier and less expensive than maternity pants. You may have to go a few sizes larger than your normal size. These pants are also great for postpartum time when you'll still have a tummy.

In the last month or two, when anything around the waist feels uncomfortable, you may want to stop wearing pants altogether. Stick to dresses or jumpers at this time.

## SKIRTS

Skirts—even maternity skirts—are not the most easily adapted items for maternity wear. However, nonmaternity drawstring skirts are often suitable for the early inflating months of pregnancy and the deflating months afterwards. Watch out for the hiked-up look in front. If your skirt's elastic waistband is too tight, simply sew a larger piece of elastic in the waistband.

Skirts may become uncomfortably binding towards the end of pregnancy. In fact, the look of skirts on pregnant women after five or six months is often peculiar. This is why we see so few in maternity wear. Occasionally you can find a pretty skirt with a matched top or one you can mix and match with different blouses during pregnancy.

## ACCESSORIES

"I never understood the importance of accessories until I got pregnant with triplets," said very pregnant Jane. "Accessories are the only part of my wardrobe which don't have to be bought at the maternity departments, and the world of interesting bags, bracelets, scarves, hats has opened right up for me."

Acessories can turn a plain and simple maternity dress into a smashing outfit. They give you a feeling of "today"—and when you're tired of wearing the same maternity dresses and tops over and over again, a change of accessories can pick up your look as well as your spirits. Be creative. Use everything from your granny's cameo brooch to your son's Indian bead pouch. Tie sashes under your belly (see Alva on p. 145), invest in a few different bags or pocketbooks, put flowers in your hair, and decorate your arms with lots of silver bracelets. Buy inexpensive necklaces, rings, etc., that are a little larger to balance your bigger shape.

A hat can be a terrific accessory. It can be whimsical and fun. Buy hats with brims large enough to balance your larger silhouette. Try an inexpensive straw hat or a cowboy hat. Borrow a man's cap or fedora. A knitted stocking cap or a soft beret are winter's best bets. Turbans or scarves artfully wrapped over a head are for the more adventurous. Five-and-ten-cent-store tennis hats look adorable in spring and summer. Splurge on accessories: they help you feel that the world of fashion is still yours while you are pregnant.

## UNDERPANTS

You may be a devotee of pretty lace-trimmed or print nylon lingerie, but think *cotton* underpants for comfort and health now that you're pregnant. They allow air to ventilate your newly sensitive vaginal area, and they're much less expensive than the designer nylon variety—which you'll appreciate when you realize how many pairs you have to buy to accommodate your changing size. Make a trip to the five-and-ten-cent store to stock up on pastel or print bikini or waist-high cotton underpants. Most women prefer the bikini underpants that do not bind the growing abdomen. These inexpensive undies are actually very cute and sexy.

## BRAS

A supporting bra with wide straps and a wide back is a must for pregnancy. Even if you're used to going without a bra, start wearing one now. Your

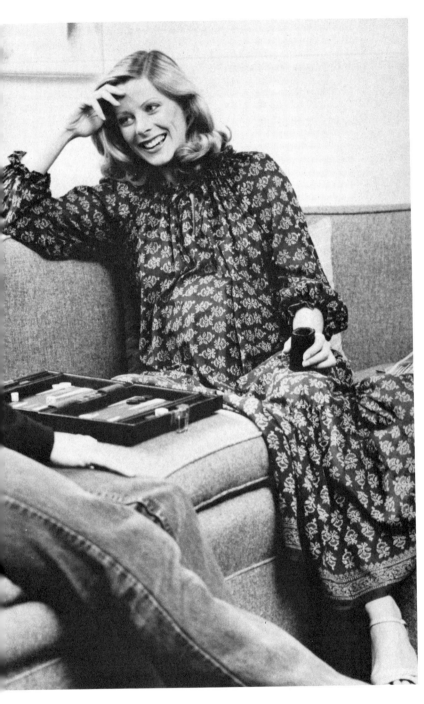

Joanne wears a nonmaternity Indian print cotton dress. Its cut is full and the fabric is light. This dress is easy to slip on for Joanne's romantic evening at home—dinner and then a game of backgammon. Wear little sandals and a pretty ribbon in your hair, and put on fresh makeup for your evening at home. Choose your at-home fashion carefully. Invest in a pretty and full bathrobe for when visitors arrive unexpectedly or for wear in the morning or evening. Caftans from the lingerie department are also great for home wear, as are many ethnic looks.

breasts are fuller and heavier from pregnancy and a good bra will save your breasts from losing muscle and skin tone. You should wear a bra twenty-four hours a day when your breasts get heavy. Try to find comfortable, well-fitting supportive cotton bras in a five-and-ten-cent store or in an inexpensive department store. Synthetic fabric bras are fine but if you tend to get hot or your breasts are leaking colostrum, you'll feel better with cotton. Cotton may also prevent dermatological problems. If inexpensive bras do not fit well, try a maternity department in a better department store or a lingerie shop specializing in bras. Try not to spend a lot of money, for your size may change a few times during pregnancy. You'll usually take one back-size or one cup-size larger by the fifth month. If you plan to nurse, you can save by buying at least one cotton nursing bra both for the end of pregnancy and for use in the hospital.

## SLIPS

Invest in either a maternity half slip (a slip with a stretch fabric abdominal area inset) or a large size half slip. Although many women try to make it without one, you'll feel better with the comfort and fit of a maternity slip. You may need only one or two half slips. Some women find maternity full slips less binding. The slip fabric is usually a synthetic rayon rather than cotton as manufacturers don't understand the difference natural fibers can make at this time. If you *do* find a cotton maternity slip, grab it.

## STOCKINGS

Pantyhose are a blessing for pregnant women. They alleviate some of the pressure on your legs and, if you've gained weight, keep your thighs separated and thus help you avoid skin irritation. When your regular size gets tight, try maternity hose, a larger size, or queen-size. The latter two are just as supportive and less expensive than the maternity pantyhose. Although garter belts and regular stockings have a certain sexy chic, they should be abandoned during pregnancy. A garter belt is too binding on the growing abdomen. If you have or tend to have varicose veins, tired legs or a job where you must stand or lift, support hose are highly recommended during your pregnancy. (For more suggestions on these special stockings, see "Varicose Veins," pp. 106–107.) Avoid knee-high hose whether you have varicose veins or not. They cut off circulation in the legs.

## GIRDLES

Normally, a pregnant woman should avoid wearing any type of girdle. However, certain medical conditions may require that you wear a maternity girdle—especially after you've had several babies. Ask your obstetrician if you should wear one. These special maternity girdles are found at maternity shops and shouldn't be confused with regular girdles.

## BATHING SUITS

"Bikinis were the only answer for me while I was pregnant last year. I'm five feet ten inches and couldn't find a one-piece that was large and long enough," said Catherine, a new mother. "At first I was a little embarrassed at the beach with such a big tummy, but then I became proud because I did look good—the rest of my body was slim. So many men told me I looked great—my husband actually got jealous."

You don't have to hide your pregnancy with tent-like bathing suits, but you may not like bikinis, or you may feel reticent about wearing one now. You may be able to wear a tank suit in a larger size, or even a leotard that gives good support—and if not, it's good news to hear that maternity bathing suits are prettier than ever. Look for the following details:

- If they have bikini pants or shorts, these shouldn't bind, but should expand as your tummy grows.

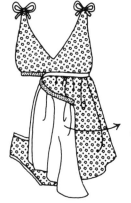

This three-piece maternity bathing suit has a Velcro fastening that enables you to remove the skirt if you want a bikini look.

- Look for a built-in bra. Or find a suit with wide shoulder straps so you can wear your own bra underneath.
- You can buy a three-piece maternity suit with a skirt that detaches under the bust line of a bikini top. This covers the bikini pants. This will give you the option of wearing a one-piece or two-piece depending on your mood or the stuffiness of your swim club!
- Make sure your top is long enough so it doesn't pull up to expose your abdomen.

## FOOTWEAR

Podiatrists, obstetricians, nurses, and others tell us medium heels (about two inches) seem to be best for pregnant women. Dr. Murray Weisenfeld, a Manhattan podiatrist, reports that flat heels tend to exaggerate the curvature of the back (already affected by the increased weight in the abdomen). High spiky heels do not provide a broad base for your foot and also increase the danger of falling.

Many pregnant women develop edema which causes swelling feet. In this case, you may have to go to the next size in shoes. Podiatrists report that many women's feet spread during pregnancy due to the added weight. They also tell us that women often experience fallen arches during pregnancy, which may require a larger shoe width as well as length. Good supportive shoes with a low heel will aid both of these conditions.

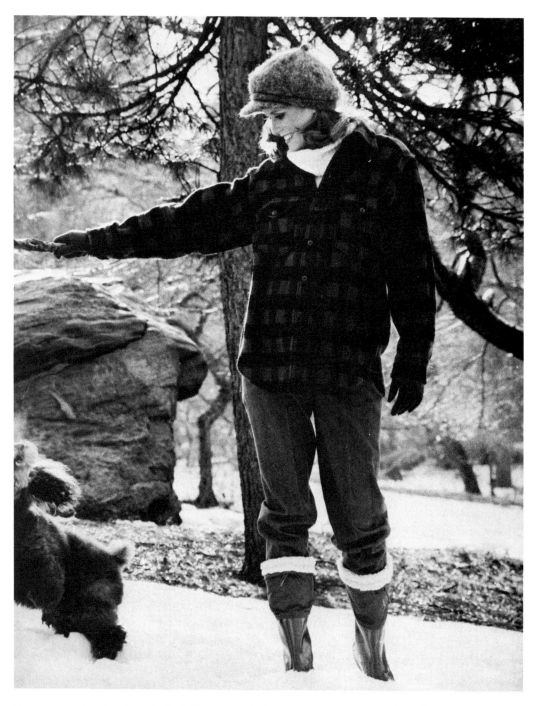

Liz borrows her husband's L. L. Bean wool shirt to wear over a turtleneck and maternity jeans. She adds her own wool cap and bright red waterproof boots to complete a great-looking outfit for play in the snow with poodle Quincy.

If you're carrying during the spring and summer, sandals may save the day and save your feet. Espadrilles and running shoes are also great footwear for pregnancy. In winter, avoid wearing your boots all day long. Keep a pair of shoes at the office to change into. If you're having trouble with your legs, avoid wearing tight boots.

## OUTDOOR WEAR

Outdoor wear is expensive and each season brings its own problems for pregnant women. Winter is perhaps the most difficult season of all. Even layers of sweaters and shells won't keep you warm in a snowstorm when your last season's winter coat doesn't close.

What can you do? We've listed seasonal solutions below, hoping that your wardrobe already contains a few of these items. The best solution during pregnancy for evening cold weather wear is the flexible cape. This is one outer wear item you may want to buy during your pregnancy. Choose a dark color so it can double for day and evening wear. Add or subtract layers of sweaters or jackets underneath as the weather grows cold or warm.

## DRESS FOR SUCCESS

The way you dress during pregnancy can make all the difference to you. Wearing pretty, well-fitting clothes during pregnancy can make you feel confident that you are admired for the lovely woman you are.

Spending time, thought, and yes, some money, on your wardrobe is going to pay off. It can make the difference between your feeling just OK or feeling like a *very special* pregnant woman.

Feeling special, pretty, and well-dressed has other benefits as well. How you feel about the way you look affects your sex life. If you dress like a frump, you may feel like one in bed. If you dress for success as a pregnant woman, these positive feelings spill over into sex—the concern of our next chapter.

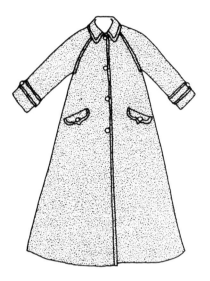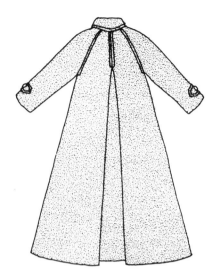

| SPRING/FALL | WINTER | SUMMER |
| --- | --- | --- |
| — Cape<br>— Shawl over other layers, such as an open blazer, etc.<br>— Wool or rain poncho, over sweater<br>— Mexican wrap sweater over your husband's turtleneck<br>— Your husband's crew neck sweater with a plaid scarf at the neck<br>— Chinese down silk jacket for evening with a long silk scarf to hide the opening | — Cape<br>— Your old winter coat with the buttons open, covered with a long pretty wool scarf<br>— A full antique fur coat from a thrift shop. This can be cut down or belted after the baby is born.<br>— Tent-style coat (see illustration above) | — Shawl<br>— Poncho<br>— Linen blazer worn open |

# CHAPTER · VI ·
## Sex and Pregnancy

TWENTY-SIX-YEAR-OLD CHRISTINE found that sex was never better than during her pregnancy. As she put it, "My sex life took off like a firecracker." This is true of many women. Some have reported experiencing their first multiple orgasm, or even the first orgasm in their lives, during pregnancy. The hormones of pregnancy often aid your sex life by causing the labia and vagina to swell and become more vascular, thus increasing their sensitivity. The swelling also results in a tighter vagina, which can make sex more pleasurable for your partner as well.

Janet, however, experienced a decreased sex drive. "Sex was okay at the very beginning, but very soon on I said 'forget it.' I had no feeling for sex at all. I accommodated my husband to some degree but for me, I just didn't like it. A few months after I had my baby I started enjoying sex again like the old days."

## THE HIGHS AND LOWS OF SEX DURING PREGNANCY

During pregnancy, most of us will not fall into the extreme categories Christine and Janet did. Most of us will be somewhere in between, diverging from our normal sexual experiences to some degree. According to Mas-

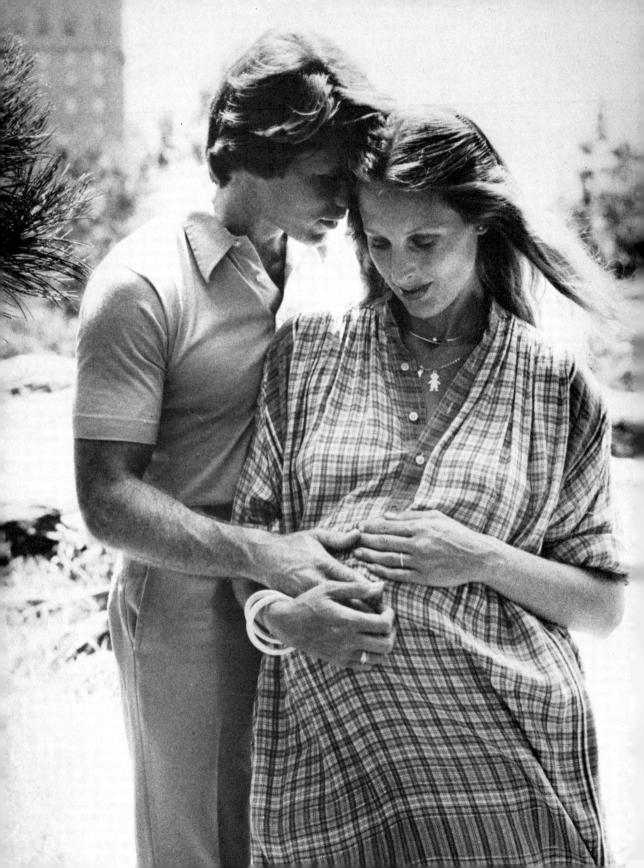

ters and Johnson, the sexual behavior authorities, one pattern of change was particularly common among pregnant women:

*First trimester*—Interest in sex decreased or was the same as before.
*Second trimester*—Interest in sex increased to a higher level than before pregnancy.
*Third trimester*—Interest in sex gradually decreased.

Different patterns have emerged in other studies. The only consistent finding about sex drive during pregnancy—according to scientific studies and among women we've interviewed—is *inconsistency*. Your sex drive may change from week to week or may stay low or high. Your taste for different kinds of sex may change as your pregnancy progresses. One study of 216 women indicates that during the first trimester most women desire vaginal stimulation but by the second and third trimester they prefer clitoral and breast stimulation.

During pregnancy each of us has a different sexual response as influenced by hormones, your or your husband's psychological makeup, physical conditions, and/or your medical condition during pregnancy. Don't compare! Listening to old wives' tales or a pregnant friend's swinging-from-the-rafters stories will do nothing but misinform and possibly make you feel inadequate. If you want a sense of the varying range of sexual experiences and emotions of pregnancy, we recommend a book called *Making Love During Pregnancy* by Elisabeth Bing and Libby Colman (New York: Bantam Books, 1977). This is one of the few books published on this important subject and it is excellent. But whatever your degree of sexual responsiveness, you may discover the one constant that seems to be common throughout pregnancy, for both you *and* your husband—this is the need to be held, the need for love.

## HOW PREGNANCY CAN CHANGE YOUR SEXUAL SELF-IMAGE

During pregnancy we have new needs for love and affection for a variety of reasons. We may fear our changed physical image makes us less attractive

Love and sex go a long way toward helping
you look and feel beautiful during pregnancy.

to our husbands. Dr. Bonnie Jacobson, a New York psychologist, says, "A pregnant image is often a distorted image of yourself. During your lifetime you get a visual image of what you and your body are like and then this image is no longer a reality. All of a sudden it's a new reality—and I think this new image and reality can make some women very uncomfortable basically."

Self-image is very important for sex. If you feel attractive and desirable, you will want and enjoy sex more. And if you are enjoying a fulfilling sex life, you'll feel more beautiful and assured.

Of course the most immediate influence on your sex life and your self-image is your husband. You may have a problem if you or your husband cannot separate affection from sexual relations. During pregnancy we feel more dependent on our husbands than ever before—physically, emotionally, and economically. We do need physical reassurance. "For many women," sayd Dr. Alfred Tanz, obstetrician at Lenox Hill Hospital, "the need for reassurance is translated into a desire for sex. For many women, the only real way men can show their love is by making love to them." Men often display the same inability to differentiate. They feel they *have* to have intercourse when hugging and caressing might be just as satisfying emotionally, and they insist on sex when the wife does not want it. When sex is a demand, on either a man or a woman, it is no fun. Men have become impotent and women disinterested in sex for precisely this reason.

Once in a while, a woman will use her pregnancy as an excuse to avoid sex. This too can be a problem. And there are some common fears women experience during pregnancy that can be extremely inhibiting.

ARE YOU AFRAID THAT:
- Your husband won't find you attractive with a big stomach?
- Your husband can hurt you or hurt the baby?
- Sex and pregnancy just don't go together?
- Your husband will take up with another woman?
- Your negative sexual experiences during pregnancy will carry over into your postpartum life?
- Your husband won't enjoy oral sex because your discharge is heavier during pregnancy?

- Your husband really doesn't love you (even though he says he does)?
- Your husband really doesn't want the baby (even though he says he does)?
- There's a third person (the baby) in bed watching you?

If you do have any of these or other fears, set a special time aside to discuss them with your husband. Letting your husband know your feelings—about your changing roles from sexy lovers to "parents" and about the financial, emotional, and other complicated changes a child brings about in your life—is yet another new task pregnancy requires of you. But what a rewarding one! The result will be a closer relationship and a feeling of security. Don't be ashamed of your doubts; no matter how serene and happy you are, you'd have to be quite simpleminded not to experience some doubts or fears at this time. Your anxieties are part of the mental groundwork that prepares you for the hectic *reality* that follows childbirth. Share them with the person you love.

## HOW *HE* FEELS . . .

Your husband's feelings and behavior during your pregnancy is crucial to the way you view yourself. Husbands often get shortchanged in pregnancy books—especially in ones such as ours which is directed solely to the woman. The emotional changes of men, and sometimes the physical changes (some men actually get nausea with their wives and one we knew gained fifteen pounds by the time his wife delivered!), can be just as dramatic.

What thoughts run through a man's mind while his wife grows larger week by week? Here is a sampling:

- What kind of father will I be? Will I be a better father than mine?
- Will I have enough money to support the baby and my wife (especially if my wife quits work to stay home with the baby full-time)?
- Will my wife give all her love and attention to the baby instead of me?

- Being married is one thing, but having a child is the biggest commitment of all.
- Can my wife get so big with the baby that she'll end up larger than me?
- Her breasts and belly are so large and her genitals so swollen that it's a little frightening.
- Will she regain her figure afterwards? Will her vagina become loose—will her breasts be different? How will that affect our sex life?
- Why is she hot and then cold? I can't keep up with her change in emotions—I'm not even sure I want to. I can play comforting husband for just so long.
- Will pregnancy hurt her health? Will she be okay? I've heard that women can die during childbirth, even today. Will the baby be okay?
- Why, just when my wife's about to give birth, do there suddenly seem to be so many sexy available women?
- I used to get a lot more attention. Everyone seems to be interested in Mary's pregnancy, and all Mary is interested in is herself. I wish I could do something creative like having a baby.

The emotions your husband experiences during your pregnancy are often new ones—ones that you and he are perhaps unprepared for. His new doubts or anxieties naturally play into your sex lives, usually negatively if you don't air them, but positively if you do. Since our culture lacks rituals which involve men in pregnancy and childbirth (prepared childbirth is slowly changing this) men often feel left out in the cold. Other cultures provide for the man's feeling of alienation during this woman-oriented time. One culture regards the man's participation as essential to the fetus's development. "New Guinea tribespeople believe that the child is nourished through intercourse," report Arthur and Libby Colman in their book *Pregnancy: The Psychological Experience* (see Bibliography). "The couple is therefore compelled to have frequent sexual relations in order to have a healthy baby."

Many men find their mates at their most irresistible during pregnancy. "I found my wife—not just all pregnant women but my wife—to be spookily attractive while she was pregnant," said Billy. "Her skin was traditionally rosy, her breasts were large, her hair was especially full and silky. She seemed to have another dimension in her personality. She seemed confident and more secure in herself than I've ever seen her. I have since read that all the hormones of pregnancy make a woman feel very serene. Her new behavior made me feel closer than ever to her. It was great for our sex life."

Another common male reaction is pride. Getting his wife pregnant is proof positive of his fertility. Jeff was particularly proud of his pregnant wife. "Nancy's doctor told her it was doubtful she could have children at all. He didn't know she'd marry *me!*"

## SEXUAL CHANGES FROM TRIMESTER TO TRIMESTER

Each of the three trimesters of pregnancy is characterized by its own set of physical, hormonal, and emotional changes—all of which contribute to new sexual attitudes and experiences. Listed below are some of the complex factors within each trimester that might heighten or decrease your interest in sex.

**First Trimester.** The most dramatic hormonal changes occur during the first trimester.

*Painful Breasts* and *Swollen Genitals.* During pregnancy, as in sex, levels of estrogen and steroids are raised and the vagina and labia become more vascular and congested. When you become sexually aroused while you are pregnant, more blood rushes to your breasts and genitals and they become more engorged. Some women complain of breast pain (although this usually passes after the first trimester) and overly sensitive genitals. On the other hand, the newly sensitive genitals can also result in great sexual excitement.

*Added Lubrication.* Due to the added hormones of pregnancy, the vagina secretes extra lubrication which makes sex especially pleasurable.

*Nausea.* Nausea, as you well know, often characterizes the first trimester. "I couldn't think about sex," said Linda. "I was so nauseous—twenty-four hours a day—that my poor husband had to do without. It got better, of course." On the other hand, some women feel that the only time they get relief from their nausea is in bed with their husbands.

*Fatigue.* Some women are so sleepy during the first trimester they lose their interest and desire for sex.

*Fear of Miscarriage.* Most miscarriages occur during the first three months of pregnancy. A history or a fear of miscarriage may inhibit a woman's desire for sex—sometimes subconsciously. Your obstetrician may ask you to refrain from sex completely if you have a history of miscarriages. (See p. 183.)

*Accepting the Pregnancy.* Unless the pregnancy's not known, of course, a couple usually comes to accept it during the first trimester. No matter how much you want the pregnancy, having a baby still takes a lot of reconciling. People with certain moral or religious backgrounds may consciously or subconsciously consider sex solely for procreation. These people may find sex during pregnancy somehow redundant. Indeed, in the entire animal kingdom only humans and primates continue to engage in sexual activity after conception.

*Reevaluating Your Relationship with Your Mother.* At the end of the first trimester, many women become preoccupied with their relationship with their mothers. They are trying to form their own mothering identities, to sort out and incorporate their mothers' positive feelings about pregnancy and child-rearing, and to expunge their mothers' negative feelings. This may affect their relationships with their husbands, too.

**Second Trimester.** Almost all the studies reported that the second trimester is a good time for eroticism and sex. Out of 101 women studied by Masters and Johnson 82 reported that sex in the second trimester was better than ever. For some women it was better even than *before* pregnancy. Why is sex particularly good in the second trimester?

*Reevaluating Your Relationship with Your Husband.* During the second trimester your emotional focus turns slowly toward your husband, away from your mother. This means increased communication and perhaps more sex.

*Changes in Genitals.* There is even more engorgement of the genitals and more lubrication as pregnancy progresses into the second trimester.

*Nausea and Fatigue.* The nausea is over, the fatigue is gone, and you're usually full of energy.

*Fear of Miscarriage.* There is not nearly so much danger of losing the baby in the second trimester.

*Physical Size.* Your abdomen is still not too large and you still feel mobile enough for active sex. This is a period during which many couples start experimenting with new positions, often resulting in lessened inhibitions—always great for sex.

*The Baby.* The baby starts kicking. You and your husband begin enjoying the feeling that the baby's OK and will soon be here, although the birth is still too far off to worry about.

**Third Trimester.** Elizabeth had gained thirty-five pounds by her seventh month and even though she was five feet eight inches, she was *large.* Crowds seemed to part as she walked down the streets of New York, "As heavy as I was, I never felt sexier and more adorable in my life. I remember wearing sexy frilly underpants—in size *extra large*—and a sexy bra for my husband. I played silly, coquettish games with him and pictured myself as a glorious earth mother. It never occurred to me that I was anything less than beautiful."

Elizabeth reported her sex life was wonderful all during pregnancy. We suspect Elizabeth had a strong self-image—a most important element for your last three months when you're probably the heaviest you've ever been in your life.

Although some women experience a gradual increase in their desire for sex right through the third trimester, most studies show a general decrease of interest in sex in the last trimester. What are the factors contributing to this decrease?

*New Focus on Self.* The focus has shifted from your mother in the first trimester, to your husband in the second, and finally to yourself in the third. As you become more self-absorbed, sex might be of little importance.

*Larger Physical Size.* Your body becomes too large and awkward for sexual gymnastics. Lovemaking sessions might be shorter.

*New Body Discomforts.* New body discomforts appear, such as Braxton-Hicks cramps (intermittent contractions of the uterus at the end of pregnancy), shortness of breath, or heartburn. All of these problems discourage sexual activity.

*Orgasm Changes.* One study shows that the rate of orgasm declines for most women in the last trimester.

*Obstetrician's Prohibition.* Your obstetrician may ask you to refrain from sex the last six weeks (see pp. 182–83). By this time you might welcome this prohibition. In the place of intercourse, you and your husband can hold and cuddle or use other methods to please and show affection for each other. Other couples continue lovemaking until the very end, enjoying petting even during labor! (But don't have intercourse or touch the vagina after your water has broken. Once the water is broken the baby is no longer protected from infection. Baths are also prohibited at this point.)

During the final period of physical awkwardness and joy/fear about the imminent birth, every woman needs attention and reassurance. Let your husband know you need it. If you don't communicate your feelings, the last trimester can be a difficult period.


## SEXUAL FEARS DURING PREGNANCY

After Mary announced her pregnancy, her husband Fred seemed less interested in sex. One night when Mary was four and a half months pregnant and her stomach had just started to show, she cuddled up to her husband and they started making love. When they got into their usual male-superior or "missionary" position, Fred tightened up. Bracing himself on his hands and knees, he entered Mary without even touching the rest of her body. Mary started to laugh. "Fred, this isn't a gym!" she said. "You don't have to do push-ups over me now that I'm pregnant." Fred was concerned that he might hurt the baby by putting pressure on Mary's abdomen. A trip to the obstetrician together cleared this up. She told them the fetus floats in a sack of water and Mary's abdomen could bear the pressure.

Many people are misinformed about sex during pregnancy. A discussion with your obstetrician could arrest problems before they start. One study showed that only ten percent of the women interviewed were told by their obstetricians about comfortable positions for sex. Dr. Don Sloan, Director of Psychosomatics at New York Medical College, Lenox Hill Hospital, reports that the most common fear of pregnant couples is that touching the woman will hurt the baby.


## FREEDOM TO EXPLORE

If you don't feel uncomfortable, and if your doctor hasn't forbidden certain positions for medical reasons, you can have sex in any position—up to a point. When your belly becomes too large and the male-superior position too uncomfortable, other positions can be used. Many couples feel that being forced to experiment with new positions during pregnancy is one of nature's gifts. Their experimentation makes them freer, and they happily continue the new positions after they've had the baby.

Before your abdomen grows too large, use your favorite sexual positions. By the fourth, fifth, or sixth months, you may want to try a few of these:

- Side by side, lying down facing each other, the woman's bottom leg under the man and the other on top. Front entry.
- Front to backside position. The same position as above, only the woman faces the opposite direction. Rear entry.
- Woman stands and bends from waist and husband, standing, enters from the rear.
- Partly sideways. The man is in the superior position, but his weight is off to the side.
- Sitting on the edge of a chair. The woman sits on a chair. The man kneels and enters her from the front.
- The woman lies on her back with legs raised on man's shoulders. He kneels and enters her from the front.
- Female-superior. Woman kneels or lies on man. This is particularly good because the woman can control the penetration.
- The woman lies on her back on a bed dangling her legs over the side. The man kneels on the floor beside the bed and penetrates from the front.

## FIVE WAYS TO MAKE YOUR SEX LIFE ROSIER

While you're experimenting with new positions, you may also explore new attitudes concerning sex. Pregnancy is a wonderful time to find new dimensions in your sexual self. Improving your sex life has other benefits too—it's the oldest and most available beauty elixir. Your pregnant glow will become even rosier. Indulge yourself!

1. Change the time of day you make love. If you work and are exhausted in the evening after dinner, switch your lovemaking to the early morning. Or, if you are lucky enough to be able to take a nap in the afternoon, you might have more energy when your husband first comes home from work.

2. Enjoy your weekends together. If this is your first baby, these may be the last weekends the two of you can enjoy alone for some time. Spend a Sunday sleeping, reading the papers, talking, making love.

3. If your sex drive has decreased, show your husband you are still interested in him and in sex by doing something out of the ordinary. Surprise him with new satin sheets, or light a candle in the bedroom and play Mozart. Or try some pretty sheer lingerie.

4. Don't compare your sex life with anybody else's. Dr. Don Sloan reminds his patients that there are no grades for sex. The only measure is receiving pleasure.

5. Keep communication open. Positions and techniques that once gave you or your husband pleasure might no longer do so as your pregnancy progresses. This can be bewildering for both of you. Talk to your husband about your feelings and encourage him to tell you his.

## EXERCISES FOR SEX

The best exercise for sex is the Kegel exercise described in Chapter IV, "Your Pregnant Body—Staying Healthy and Fit." Tell your husband about it, so you can practice it in bed! You'll learn about Kegels in prepared-childbirth class but you'll want to start the exercise earlier in pregnancy.

To practice Kegel exercises, tighten up your vaginal muscles while your husband's penis is inside you. Try to distinguish these muscles from the abdominal and buttocks muscles and do not tighten the latter two. Do this a few times. Ask your husband to gauge your progression. Repeat several times during your lovemaking sessions.

A well-toned pregnant body is a real plus for sex during pregnancy—so keep up with the exercise program you've developed to achieve good muscle tone and more vigor. Exercising also produces energy—one element very necessary for a good sex life, especially during late pregnancy. Exercise, eat well, and sleep sufficiently. All these disciplines aid good sex during pregnancy.

## WHEN SEX IS PROHIBITED

When Patty was four months pregnant, she and her husband Dirk were watching a comedy show about a very pregnant woman and her husband. The woman on TV returned home from the doctor and announced to her husband that they couldn't have sexual relations until after the baby was born. The audience laughed knowingly, but Dirk's jaw dropped. "Do we have to stop sex?" Dirk said incredulously.

Fortunately for Dirk, times have changed. Patty and Dirk's obstetrician told them they could continue sex until Patty's water broke. However, some doctors are still conservative about sex during pregnancy, and advise women to stop having intercourse six weeks before their due date. The two reasons for this are the possibility of a vaginal infection and the possible rupture of the placenta in the case of a placenta previa (see the Glossary at the back of the book). It would be best to follow your own obstetrician's advice on this matter. Discuss any questions with her.

Orgasm is usually allowed even if your doctor prohibits intercourse in the last six weeks. Masturbating is allowed—as long as nothing enters the vagina. Oral sex is another alternative. But your partner should *never* blow or force air into your vagina. The air can travel from the vagina through to the endocervical canal into the vascular system. This air can then travel to the brain and cause a fatal air embolism.

## WHY SOME WOMEN HAVE TO GIVE UP SEX

There are medical conditions in the presence of which your doctor may ask you to avoid sexual intercourse or even orgasm during certain periods of your pregnancy. He might even ask you to avoid intercourse all the way through pregnancy.

Doctors prohibit sex when bleeding during intercourse makes them suspect a placenta previa. Spotting can also occur after sexual intercourse even when there is no placenta previa because the vagina is more vascular and more susceptible to bleeding. This is usually no cause for concern, although you should report it to your doctor. The bleeding susceptibility usually passes.

If you have a past history of miscarriages, your obstetrician may suggest avoiding sex, especially during the first three or four months. Or, if you have a history of premature delivery, or are expecting twins or triplets, sex may be prohibited toward the end of pregnancy. This is because orgasm can produce uterine contractions which may bring on labor. It is also believed that the hormone prostaglandin, present in semen, may bring on labor.

What can your husband do for you if intercourse and orgasm are off limits for any length of time during your pregnancy? Your partner can:

- Slowly undress you and give you a body massage with a moisturizing lotion.
- Massage your back, legs, and arms with a sudsy washcloth in the shower.
- Hold and caress you.
- Massage your feet. Very sensual and pleasing.
- Tell you how much he loves you.
- Wash your hair and comb it.
- Give you a facial massage with a rich moisturizer.
- Smooth scented body oil over your body.
- Just touch your cheek.

## THE JOY OF PREGNANT SEX

Luckily for us, medical thinking allows us more sexual freedom during pregnancy than ever before. If our pregnancies are healthy and normal, we can continue our sex lives as they were and even discover something new.

Sex plays a very important role during pregnancy. It aids you emotionally, soothing and relaxing an anxious mother-to-be.

For most of us, expecting a baby provides a new romantic dimension to our sex lives. Considering that sex has been almost overliberated in the last few decades, many women we interviewed felt that the anticipation, excitement, and pride of pregnancy restored or recreated romance within their marriages. A new body awareness emerged as both men and women became fascinated with the woman's pregnant body. Couples smiled when they related how a new warmth emerged as they lay in bed and caressed the woman's big stomach, waiting for the baby's movements. As they watched the result of their physical love grow day by day, their love for each other deepened and sex became even more fulfilling.

# CHAPTER · VII ·
# *Your Hospital Stay*

MANY OF US FEEL REMARKABLY ENERGIZED toward the end of pregnancy—like the woman who told us, "I worked a full day, went home, began labor and delivered that night." This energy may come from your subconscious (you know you will soon give birth), or your system, which has possibly been given a final hormonal jolt.

On the other hand, you may also feel exhausted these last few weeks. Working or even making the evening meal becomes so tiring you may want only to lie down in bed and watch TV.

One instinct all of us seem to feel is the urge to nest. During our final period of pregnancy we scrub our homes, recheck the nursery for the fifteenth time for every detail needed, practice our Lamaze breathing, and stock the refrigerator with more frozen dinners and other food than our husbands could eat in a month. While you're in this mood, make sure the suitcase you're taking to the hospital contains the items below. Pack your prettiest! This is one of the most important times of your life. Play it up. Look and feel lovely as a brand-new mother.

*Suitcase Checklist*
- [ ] *2 to 4 nightgowns.* Wear the gown the hospital gives you for the night following the baby's birth, so you won't stain your own with blood

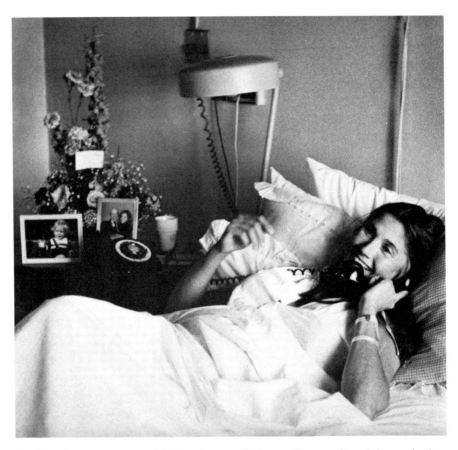

Gail, a thirty-six-year-old first-time mother, two hours after delivery feels too excited to sleep. "It's a girl," she tells the world.

and the discharge that follows childbirth. Change into your own wash-and-wear or cotton button-down nightgown in the morning. If you plan to nurse, button-down nightgowns make things much simpler. Hospital gowns are difficult to nurse in since they usually tie in the back. Save your prettiest satin or frilly cotton nightgown for visitors or your husband.

☐ *1 pretty bedjacket.*

☐ *1 bathrobe.* A floor-length washable robe which cannot be seen through makes you feel comfortable and looks well when receiving visitors or going to newborn and nursing classes at the hospital.

☐ *1 pair of slippers.* Backless slippers that are easy to slide into are handy and are especially helpful for women who have had Caesarean section deliveries.

☐ *Bras.* Pack 2 nursing bras if you plan to breast-feed your baby. Bring 1 or 2 snug-fitting bras if you don't plan to nurse.

☐ *Underpants.* Bring your cotton maternity underpants so that if they get stained, you can simply throw them out.

☐ *2 sanitary belts.* The one-inch-wide bikini-type belt works well since it doesn't cut into your full abdomen the way the slimmer type may.

☐ *A loose-fitting going-home outfit for yourself and clothes for the baby.* For yourself, a full dress is perhaps less discouraging than pants and a top—you can't count on fitting into your prepregnancy clothes immediately. For the baby, pack a cap, a stretchy or pretty nightgown, and a warm blanket. You'll also need 2 or 3 cloth diapers, a T-shirt, and a sweater. The key is to bring the proper clothes for the weather.

## LOOKING YOUR BEST

Both you and your baby will be on view at the hospital. *You* can do something about the way you look. Take advantage of all the help beauty products afford. Pamper and beautify yourself with the following:

*Beauty Survival Kit*
☐ Makeup, including clear lip gloss (Pack in a small cosmetic bag.)
☐ Makeup mirror
☐ Moisturizer
☐ Body lotion
☐ Special skin care products
☐ Spray bottle of mineral water
☐ Small pack of tissues
☐ Perfume
☐ Toothbrush and toothpaste
☐ Razor
☐ Deodorant

*For Your Hair*

☐ Shampoo and conditioner (Buy your favorites in small trial-size bottles or transfer your shampoo and conditioner to small plastic bottles.)

☐ Electric rollers and/or portable hand blow-dryer (Check with your hospital to make sure they allow these.)

☐ Small box or pretty tin to hold new hair ribbons, bobby pins, combs, barrettes, covered rubber bands

☐ Comb and brush

☐ Shower cap

## OTHER NEEDS

If you have taken prepared-childbirth classes, you'll be needing your "Lamaze bag." Your prepared-childbirth instructor will give you a list of what this bag should contain—contents often vary from class to class. Pack this bag separately since you'll be needing it during labor. Here are some other items you may need:

☐ Camera

☐ Film (Black-and-white Tri-X film does not require a flash.)

☐ Flash (Check to see whether your hospital permits this.)

☐ Personal phone book, a list of must-calls, and a roll of dimes

☐ Magazines and books

☐ Eyeglasses, if you wear them

☐ Thank-you postcards, stamps, pen

☐ Champagne, wine, mineral water, or soda (for celebrating after the baby is born)

Do not bring your good jewelry, a large amount of money, or other valuables to the hospital. The hospital can usually lock up money or valuables, but it is wiser to leave them at home. Never keep your good things in the hospital room. If they are stolen, the hospital will not be responsible for them. Do bring change for newspapers and little goodies.

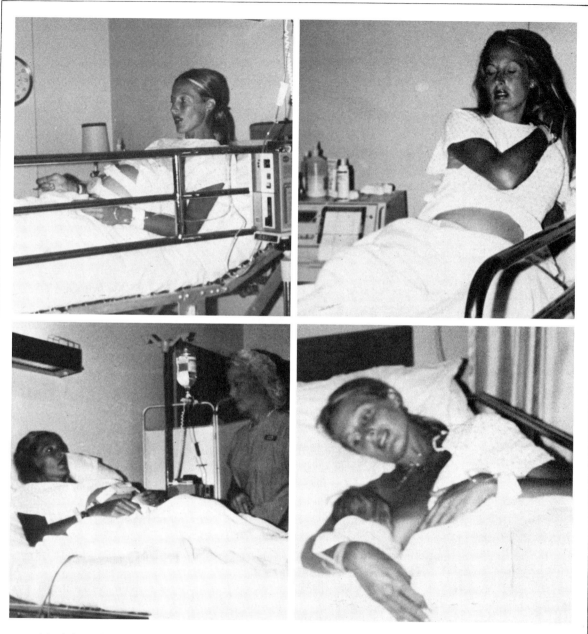

Madolin's husband took pictures during the labor. This was her third child, and with the help of prepared childbirth Madolin was confident and relaxed. In the last picture Madolin nurses newborn Kier.

Make sure your husband or helper brings your insurance identification card and a check to the hospital with you. Many hospitals will not admit a patient until the financial paperwork is completed. Your checking-in will be speedier if you have all the necessary documents in hand.

EIGHT WAYS TO BRIGHTEN UP YOUR HOSPITAL ROOM

The legend goes that Ethel Kennedy never went to have her babies (all eleven of them) without her Porthault linen sheets. Pretty bed linen is a wonderful idea for every new mother. Your hospital stay can be immeasurably brightened by adding your personal touch to an otherwise dull and depressing hospital room. You can surprise a friend by decorating her room for her as a gift. If you share a semiprivate room, you can decorate your side of the room or your night table and wall. Here are some ideas:

1. Bring your own favorite floral print or monogrammed *top* sheets and pillowcases. Use a top sheet *only* since you might stain a bottom sheet. You might also want to bring your most luxurious towels from home. Take care not to lose your linens in the hospital wash!
2. Use a pretty blanket cover or quilt for your hospital bed.
3. Decorate your hospital bed with small pillows—eyelet pillows, a heart-shaped pillow, a cat-shaped pillow, a sachet pillow.
4. Place a pretty framed picture of your family on your bedside table. Have a Polaroid picture taken of you with your baby, your husband, your mother, or a special friend and display it on your table. You'll treasure these pictures later.
5. Use a fabric-covered sewing box or decorative tin to hold everything that accumulates on the hospital bedside table.
6. Bring a clock, radio, cassette recorder (to play your favorite music), or TV if your hospital doesn't provide rentals.
7. We know one husband who brought his wife's favorite rocking chair up to her room for nursing!

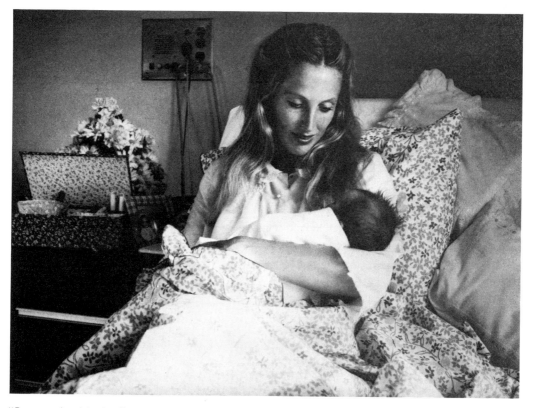

"For my third baby," says Madolin, "I decided I wanted my prettiest things surrounding me while I recuperated in the hospital. I wanted my favorite sheets, pillows, pictures, even my covered sewing box full of my makeup and nail polish."

8. You'll probably get loads of flowers. Don't keep them all piled on one table. Spread the bouquets around the room, on windowsills, even on the floor. Save one flower to dry from each bouquet. Then combine these flowers for a potpourri remembrance of your baby's birth.

## LOOKING GOOD FOR THE BIG MOMENT

"I had it all planned," said Agnetta, a great-looking blonde. "Four days before my due date, I was booked into a plush salon for an entire workover. I was going to have my hair done, get a facial, a manicure and pedicure. I wanted to look as cool and glamorous as possible when I had my baby."

Nature intervened and Agnetta started labor a week early. "I caught a glimpse of myself going out the door to the hospital and screamed," she said. " 'Look at my hair—let me go back and wash it!' I begged my husband. He was having no part of that and off we went with hair, nails, and face undone. I was more upset about my appearance than my labor pains!"

It may sound frivolous, but almost every woman we spoke to was very concerned about the way she would look for labor and the delivery of her baby. We don't consider it vanity; it probably has more to do with esthetics and control. For in the minds of most women, having a baby is a spiritual and challenging episode rather than a medical event. One woman said that if she felt she looked clean, pretty, and pulled together—in control of her looks—she would feel more in control of the birth.

Here are some beauty preparations you can make when labor begins, *if* your contractions are mild, and *if* your doctor tells you you have time:

- Take a shower and wash your hair. Baths are not permitted after the membranes rupture, releasing the amniotic fluid.
- Blow dry your hair. If need be, ask your husband to help. Curl your hair with electric rollers if you like.
- Pull your hair back off your face with a pretty ribbon or combs. Keep these accessories in a special place so you can find them easily at this point!
- After you've cleaned your face, apply a light moisturizer. Do not apply foundation, blusher, gleamer, etc. Doctors and nurses want to see your own color, not Revlon's.
- Make sure your nails are free of colored nail polish.
- Keep a spray bottle of mineral water in your refrigerator to give yourself a refreshing spritz when you feel hot and perspiry as you labor at home. When you leave for the hospital, throw this into your Lamaze bag for use in the labor room. Since most women feel very hot during labor, this cool spray helps enormously. Pack handkerchiefs to pat off the water.

- Don't wear jewelry to the hospital since the nurses will only remove it. Most women are allowed to wear their wedding band, however.
- Apply clear lip gloss and reapply it as it comes off. Lip gloss helps keep your lips from becoming dry during labor.

## NOW THAT YOU'VE HAD YOUR BABY— POSTPARTUM ACHES AND PAINS

From the moment you deliver your baby until six weeks after, your hormones, body, and emotions undergo a change more radical and violent than anything you have experienced before. The period is called "puerperium" and includes the involution (or return to the normal, nonpregnant state) of the uterus, abdominal wall, skin, body fluid distribution, and other parts of the body.

Euphoria is usually all you feel at first after you have your baby. The following morning, however, the aches and pains of giving birth are there to greet you along with the morning sun. When your nurse brings your breakfast tray, she may hear a loud "ouch" as you sit up for coffee and eggs. Of all the postpartum complaints of a vaginal birth, nurses tell us that sore bottoms are most common. This discomfort in the perineum is caused by the episiotomy stitches and/or hemorrhoids, the latter often causing the most pain.

EPISIOTOMY. The soreness you feel in your perineum will depend to a large degree on the size of your episiotomy incision. Women who have small babies—and therefore small episiotomies—feel less discomfort than women who had large episiotomies. The length of your labor and the difficulty of the delivery are also factors in how your perineum will feel after the birth.

The most important factor in caring for your sore bottom is cleanliness. After you urinate or have a bowel movement, *blot* rather than wipe your perineum from front to back being careful not to disturb your stitches. Many hospitals provide a "peri-bottle" or "squeegy bottle." This is filled with warm tap water and is sprayed on the perineal area after voiding. It feels very soothing. Or, apply witch hazel compresses, often provided by the hospital, to your stitches.

When you take a shower, use a sudsy washcloth to bathe the perineum. Some women prefer lathering this area with their bare hands to investigate the episiotomy and any hemorrhoids that may have occurred during delivery. A gentle massage of the perineum encourages the circulation and speeds the healing process.

The first treatment for a sore perineum is to apply gauze-covered ice to the area. The cold is used to prevent and/or decrease swelling and edema. After twelve hours, heat should be applied to aid circulation and encourage healing. Your hospital may provide one or all of the following treatments for the perineal area:

*Topical anesthetic cream.* This is applied to the stitches to numb the area and reduce pain.

*Sitz bath.* This is a small portable basin which fits on the toilet seat. Warm water flows onto the perineal area to soothe and encourage healing.

*Perineal heat lamp.* Your perineal area is exposed to this lamp for a few minutes once or twice a day to encourage healing.

HEMORRHOIDS. If you pushed out hemorrhoids along with the baby, or you had them before, they're bound to be painful at this point. All the above treatments aid in soothing these swollen rectal veins. If you have been provided with a topical anesthetic for your episiotomy, apply it after each bowel movement or whenever these veins feel sore. As we said in the "Body and Exercise" chapter, you are encouraged to tuck these hemorrhoids back inside the rectum while applying the ointment or while in the shower. Do your Kegel exercises often—especially after a bowel movement—to promote healing of the hemorrhoids.

In addition, make use of every comfort or amenity the hospital can provide. Many women don't realize what they're entitled to or what's available at their hospitals to make their stay more comfortable. At the price you pay, don't be one bit shy about asking for whatever you'd like. Here are some of the services that are usually offered at hospitals:

> Sanitary pads for your personal hygiene
> Ice packs
> Sitz baths
> Heat lamps
> Sponge baths for Caesarean sections
> Pain-killers and sleeping pills
> Footstool
> Baby care class
> Breast-feeding class
> Hairdresser or manicurist working in the hospital
> TV rental
> Cart selling candy, newspapers, magazines, etc.
> Book cart
> Crafts projects
> Snacks and fruit juice
> Priest, minister, or rabbi on call

LOCHIA. Another source of discomfort in the perineal area may be the lochia, or blood from the site in the uterus where the placenta breaks away. This bleeding helps heal the uterus, and it also carries away residual material. It is usually bright red for the first two to four days, when it is called "lochia rubra."

You'll probably have to wear two "maternity" or hospital sanitary pads right after you've had your baby. Change these pads often to feel fresh and comfortable. Shower frequently. Use a peri-bottle to keep your pubic hairs from getting matted. Walk around as soon as possible—this helps the uterus involute more quickly, and shortens the duration of the lochia rubra.

ELIMINATION. Nurses encourage new mothers to void four to eight hours after birth. If you have trouble urinating the first time, try urinating in a sitz bath or in a warm shower.

The first bowel movement is often dreaded—the thought of bearing down on hemorrhoids and stitches sends many mothers racing back to their beds. Try to drink plenty of fluids, eat lots of fruits and vegetables, and take walks often. If you can't go by the third day, your doctor may prescribe a mild laxative, suppository, or enema.

AFTERPAINS. Many women are surprised to feel abdominal pains after they have the baby. These are called "afterpains" and are caused by the actively contracting uterus. These pains are felt especially sharply while nursing, because the baby's sucking releases the hormone oxytocin which starts lactation but also stimulates the contraction of the uterus.

Afterpains may last for as long as seven days but usually disappear after three. Ask your nurse for an analgesic for the pains. Lying on your stomach also helps. A full bladder elevates the uterus, causing it to work harder to contract, so urinate as often as possible.

ENGORGEMENT. Between the third and fifth day postpartum your breasts may become engorged, or uncomfortably swollen with excess milk and fluids. Frequent nursing helps this condition. You can also ask your nurse for a breast pump if necessary. Use a good supportive bra and apply heat or ice packs after you nurse to prevent the breasts from swelling after they've been emptied. Ask for a mild analgesic if you feel discomfort.

*Note for Nonnursing Mothers.* Many hospitals today avoid giving lactation-suppressing medication. They advise simply binding the breasts with a snug bra or taking a towel, wrapping it around your chest and pinning it down the front so the breasts are flat and milk cannot come in. If your breasts are uncomfortable, put ice packs on them and take aspirin to relieve any pain. Hormones, often given in the past to suppress lactation are, for the most part, not used now because of risk factors.

CAESAREAN DELIVERY. Donna, a thirty-year-old mother we interviewed who'd had a Caesarean delivery, noticed that all the "C-section" women in the hospital looked worn, pale, and disheveled while the women who'd had a natural delivery looked cheery. "They all had on makeup and had combed their hair and looked as though they cared," she said. "We all looked as if we'd just come in from a battle."

If you're one of the more than twelve percent of women giving birth who've had a Caesarean section, you'll experience more postpartum discomfort and won't be as chipper as a woman who has had a vaginal delivery and was completely awake throughout. You may have nausea, headaches, severe gas pains, and soreness at the incision. You will be on intravenous fluids for a while. Ask the nurse to put the I.V. in your right hand if you are a lefty or vice versa.

You should pamper yourself to some degree at this time, but try to get up as soon as permissible to aid your recovery. (Be sure there is someone in the room to help you get out of bed for the first days.) Ask your nurse for frequent sponge baths. They are wonderfully refreshing and give you a great lift.

When the nurse brings your baby for you to hold, be sure that your incision is covered by a pillow on your lap. Be careful not to hold the baby directly on your incision. This can be quite painful. If you are breast-feeding, ask the nurse to show you comfortable nursing positions for the Caesarean-section mother.

POSTPARTUM DEPRESSION. Everyone has heard of the postpartum depression that many women suffer after giving birth. This depression is caused by the hormonal changes of puerperium and/or other underlying psychological problems. (See pp. 324-25 for additional information.) Some postpartum blues begin one or two days after birth and last just a short while in the hospital. One friend swore that a glass of champagne with her husband every evening buoyed her spirits and helped her through her two-day postpartum blues. Another woman from Texas said she was depressed until she received two gifts—both for *her* and not the baby. One was a basket filled with nail polish, nail file, tweezers, body lotion, postcards, stamps, pen, a baby-tears plant, and magazines. The other was a pair of diamond stud earrings from her husband. (Expensive but effective therapy!) If you find yourself very depressed during your stay in the hospital, speak to your obstetrician or hospital psychiatrist. Communicate your feelings to your husband. He may be able to help immediately by providing understanding and support.

SIX POSTPARTUM EXERCISES FOR THE HOSPITAL STAY. You can start Kegel exercises on the delivery table after the baby's been born! If you haven't had a Caesarean section, the rest of the exercises listed below will help you regain your energy, muscle tone, vigor, and start you on the road to getting back into shape. Women who have had Caesareans should check with their doctor before doing *any* exercise.

### 1st day

1. Lie on your tummy. (These are definitely not for Caesarean section deliveries.)
2. Lie down or stand up and do deep abdominal breathing. Place your hand on your abdomen and feel your stomach expand as you take a deep breath. Slowly exhale. Repeat 5 times.
3. Continue your Kegel exercises. Tighten and release the vagina ten times whenever you think of it.

### 2nd day

4. Lie flat on your back. Lift head so your chin touches your chest and flex your feet. Lower head and point toes. Repeat 10 times.
5. Head roll. Sit up in your bed keeping your back straight. Roll your head gently around starting at the front, then the side, then back and front. Repeat 3 times in one direction and then reverse.
6. Shoulder roll. Rotate your shoulders forward 4 times and 4 times back. Continue these exercises throughout your hospital stay.

## FIVE GOODIES TO SMUGGLE PAST THE NURSE

Systems and institutions are no fun if you can't knock them. This goes doubly for hospitals. Have fun and be a little naughty. Here are some suggestions:

1. *Drink.* Have your husband smuggle in champagne, wine, beer (great for nursing mothers!), or soda along with plastic glasses to serve guests. Have fruit, cookies, or nuts for your guests and throw a little party when they visit. Don't tire yourself out, though. Limit your guests if you find you're getting too little rest.
2. *Food.* In place of a hospital lunch, have your husband bring you your favorite meal. Try some smoked salmon, black bread, cucumber salad, and a luscious strawberry tart as a special treat. A local Italian restaurant sent Catherine, a thirty-three-year-old first-time mother, her favorite Italian dinner—spaghetti marinara, tossed green salad, Italian

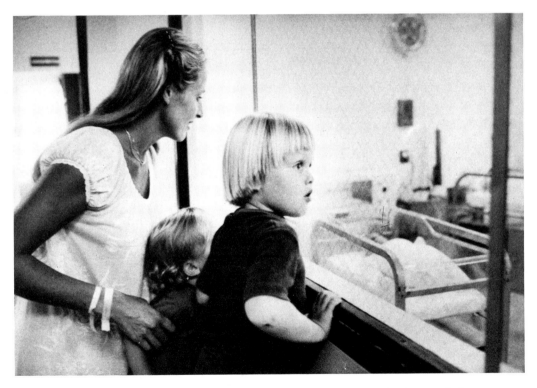

Devon and Palin visit their mother and new baby sister, Kier, at the hospital. Says Madolin, "I could relax and enjoy the baby once I saw the boys."

bread, cheese, and rum cake—as a baby gift. Have your favorite restaurant send over a special meal complete with tray, linen, glass, and silverware.

3. *Your hairdresser* (if he or she is willing). Only your own hairdresser knows exactly how you like your hair done.

4. *Your children.* Many hospitals today allow children to come to the lounge of the maternity floor to visit with their mother and/or the new baby. If your hospital doesn't allow children, ask your doctor if she can make special arrangements for your child to visit. One woman we know sneaked down to the lobby to see her five-year-old son every night.

5. *Your husband.* Close the door to your room or pull the curtain (if you have a semiprivate room) so you can have some time alone to yourselves.

## TIME-SAVING TIPS

Although your days in the hospital will be filled with visitors, meals, your baby, classes, telephoning, etc., there are snatches of time here and there you can utilize. You'll be amazed at how little time you will have at home to do these chores—so use your spare time now.

- When you receive flowers or a gift in the hospital, jot down a quick thank-you on a post card and send it off *immediately.* Thank-you duties pile up very quickly.

- Address birth anouncements. If you're having special announcements printed, ask the printer for the envelopes in advance so that you can address them during your hospital stay.

- If you're planning a party to celebrate your baby's birth, make a list of friends you'd like to invite. When you talk to them on the phone or write them thank-you notes, mention the date and time of the party too. This will save you the trouble of sending out separate invitations.

- Many baby books have chapters on the first week of life. Read a little every day. This will give you information so you'll have an idea about what to ask the pediatrician when he visits.

Your husband can also help you with the following:

- Call the baby nurse, housekeeper, or whoever is coming to help you. Tell them the time and date they are expected.
- Call the diaper service, drug store (to order disposable diapers, formula, etc.) and tell them when to start delivery.
- Arrange for the housekeeper, your mother, your husband, or a good friend to clean and straighten up your house before you get home from the hospital. There's nothing worse than walking into a messy home.

## GOING HOME

When you leave the hospital make sure you look your best. Wear a pretty dress and take the time to do your makeup and hair. If you live in a city, hire a limousine to take you home in style. Take lots of pictures and *savor* this special day. One of the great dramas of your life is over, and another is about to begin—your motherhood. It's all still very exciting and the changes do not end here—there will be more.

# CHAPTER ·VIII·
# Your Body Postpartum

THE FEMALE BODY IS A REMARKABLE MACHINE. It seems somehow able to shrug off the enormous changes of pregnancy and the physical drama of birth: many of the problems which arise during pregnancy correct or modify themselves within weeks after delivery; and bodily complaints such as varicose veins and hemorrhoids, which are aggravated by pregnancy, improve immediately after the pressure of the baby is gone. Although we may not be as hearty as primitive women we hear of—women who squat in the fields, deliver, and return to their hoeing with the baby at breast—most women today pride themselves on staying fit, strong, and well-educated for childbirth and a quick recovery.

Of course some of the problems of pregnancy still need extra attention. New problems may also arise during your first six weeks postpartum. New mothers have asked: "How can I relieve the soreness of my episiotomy now that I'm at home?" "Is there any way to get rid of hemorrhoids—permanently?" "What can I do about the discoloration of my varicose veins?" "Will breast-feeding ruin the look of my breasts?"

You may share Karen's feelings about herself. Standing and appraising herself in front of the mirror, she said, "It looks like I've got more baby fat than my little Melissa. What exercising and dieting I've got to do to get

Joanne, six weeks postpartum here, is happy to have her body back to herself. Joanne is one of those lucky "elastic bands" whose figures snap right back into shape.

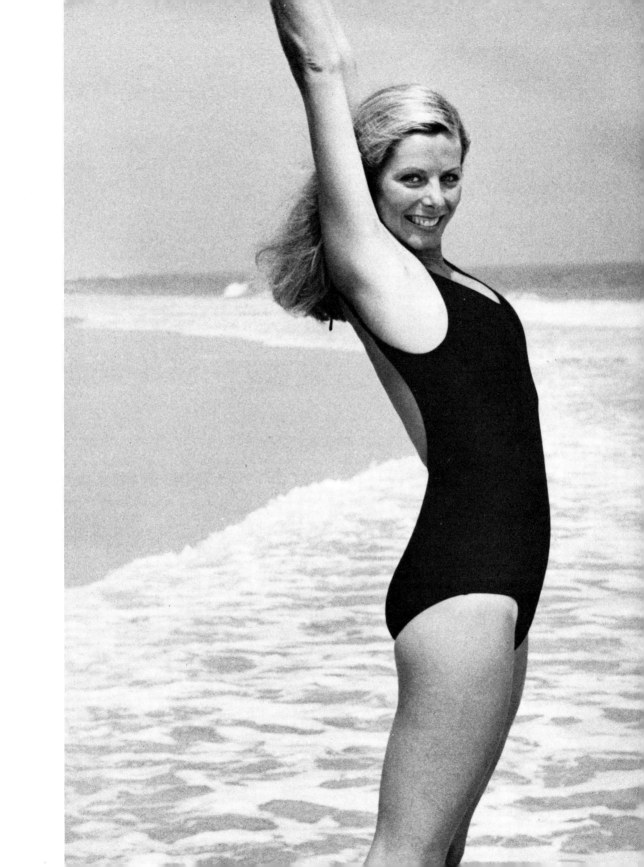

back into shape! The thought of it right now while I'm so tired is just hopeless."

It can all seem overwhelming when you take a good look at yourself upon arriving home from the hospital. You've still got a sizable abdomen, your breasts may be swollen with milk if you're nursing, and the rest of you is still quite a distance from your glorious slimmest. But to judge your body shortly after you have a baby is unfair. You'll be losing inches and pounds happily for the next month and a half without dieting or exercising while your body involutes.

But even after these six weeks you may still be overweight, and your body may look very different to you than it did before you got pregnant. What bodily changes does pregnancy bring about? Why do different parts of the body take longer than others to regain their shape and strength? Why is it so hard to lose some fat deposits after the baby is born? To what extent can exercise modify postpartum figure problems? Which exercises should you avoid at this time?

These are only some of the questions you may have about your body when you get home from the hospital. Don't ignore them. Care for your body and your looks during this period is essential—just when you find that the baby is taking up twenty-three of the twenty-four hours in a day. If you don't look and feel your best, how can you do your best? Don't overextend yourself during this period. Find out what in fact is happening to you and why, and then work *with* your body, without overstraining and pushing yourself, to get it back in shape. Proper care will speed you on the road to recovery and help you look and feel like a healthy new mother.

## PERINEAL CARE

The most obvious and immediate changes in your body take place in the perineal area, especially if—like most of us—you have had an episiotomy. By the time you get home, your episiotomy may have already healed. Synthetic catgut is usually used for episiotomy stitches. This catgut dissolves or falls out, often within a few days; and most women heal naturally within six to ten days after delivery. To speed the healing process and make yourself feel clean and more comfortable, especially during the first six weeks of recovery, try these simple steps:

- If your stitches are very uncomfortable, continue to use an anesthetic ointment obtained at the hospital.
- Take a homemade "sitz bath." Fill your bathtub with two or three inches of warm water and sit in it for a few minutes. Keep it shallow so water will not enter your vagina (which might cause infection). The warm water will soothe and stimulate circulation in the area, and it feels wonderful.
- When you're taking a shower, face away from the spray and bend over to let the warm water run over the perineal area. Make sure the force of the water is gentle and don't let the water hit the stitches directly. This may hurt.
- Spray on fresh warm water from a peri-bottle (see pp. 193–94) after eliminating or whenever you feel uncomfortable. Pat dry with toilet tissue.
- Don't cushion this area too much. The inflated tubes that are often given to new mothers in the hospital for sitting are not recommended for at-home use. The area must be stimulated to some degree by its normal contact with the surfaces of chairs and sofas.
- Do your Kegel exercises.

## LOCHIA

When you leave the hospital you will still be wearing a sanitary napkin to absorb the lochia—which at this stage will be the light pink "lochia serosa" not the bright red "lochia rubra" you had in the hospital. During the four to six weeks it usually takes for this lochia to completely subside, the flow may stop for a day or two and then start up again, much like a menstrual period.

Lochia normally has a unique odor—something like bleaching liquid, as one woman described it—and this may mix with your perspiration, making you feel less than fresh and clean. To deal with this:

- Shower frequently or sit in a warm sitz bath.
- Spray your arms and neck with a lightly scented cologne after showering, or use a perfumed body lotion after you shower. These lotions last and last.
- Change your sanitary pad each time you go to the bathroom even if you don't need to. It will make you feel cleaner and more comfortable. Use minipads when the flow is less.
- Try wearing cotton underpants and adhesive pads rather than a belt with its nonadhesive sanitary pad. They're more comfortable. Do not use a tampon at this time; wait until your doctor gives you the okay.

| MEDICAL ALERT | EXCESSIVE BLEEDING |
|---|---|

A sudden flow of bright red lochia usually indicates you are trying to do too much and have opened up blood vessels that should be healing. Call your obstetrician if the blood is bright red and flowing copiously (more than one pad per hour over six hours). Do as little as possible for a few days and rest frequently.

The passing of blood clots from the vagina is scary to someone who has never experienced it before, but it usually means nothing. These clots, having accumulated during the night's sleep are usually passed upon getting up in the morning. Large clots or any passed tissues (whitish in color) should be reported to your obstetrician.

Another warning signal of trouble is a strong offensive odor from the lochia or from vaginal discharge. This indicates an infection and your obstetrician should be notified.

## DOUCHING

Douching is not recommended at all since the vagina is self-cleaning. Nature does exquisite work, keeping all parts of the body clean.

If you do prefer to douche, wait until your doctor gives you the okay. You are usually allowed to resume douching when you resume sexual intercourse, about four to six weeks after delivery.

## HEMORRHOIDS

Whether you pushed out hemorrhoids during delivery, developed them during pregnancy, or had them before and saw them worsen with pregnancy, these mean and troublesome clusters of swollen veins in the rectum will probably recede significantly within six weeks. In the interim they can make you feel very uncomfortable.

Try warm baths, commercial hemorrhoid medication, Kegel exercises, and witch hazel pads for relief. (Also see pp. 117–18.) If hemorrhoids persist for more than two to three months and cause pain, bleeding, or itch, speak to your doctor. Itching can be caused by fecal leakage and should be treated by a proctologist.

There are many ways to treat severe hemorrhoids, including injecting, freezing, or having them surgically removed. A method that is gaining popularity is the rubber band technique. It's a low cost, relatively painless way to remove hemorrhoids and can be performed as an out-patient procedure. A rubber band is applied around the base of the hemorrhoidal tissues. The blood supply is then cut off. Within three or four days, the tissue dies. This is generally considered a better alternative than surgery, which is not indicated as often as it once was.

## THE PELVIC FLOOR

Kegel exercises (see pp. 118–20) are even more important *now* than during pregnancy since the pelvic floor muscles have been stretched during delivery. One young woman just home from the hospital complained that every time she stood up she felt "like everything was going to fall out." Her obstetrician ordered her to do Kegel exercises to recover the strength of these tired muscles.

Besides other benefits mentioned in other chapters, Kegel exercises will help with the following:

- You'll be able to control urine and aid in bowel movement by increasing muscle control over the perineal area.
- You'll be able to regain your pelvic floor *support*. By contracting your pelvic floor each time you get up from a chair or bed, you'll avoid the achy feeling our young mother complained of.
- Doing Kegel exercises helps alleviate or prevent such problems as a prolapsed uterus. It is also necessary to get these muscles back into shape before you have your next child. Don't let this area grow weaker by misuse. Start your Kegel exercises now!

## WHAT PREGNANCY HATH WROUGHT

Your abdominal muscles have been hit harder than any part of your body during pregnancy. They have been stretched to twice their length while carrying the baby. They involute for six weeks after birth and will be close to their original length by three months. Good, hard exercise, however, is required to bring them back to their original length.

Most postpartum exercise classes put special emphasis on regaining your abdominal strength. This is especially important for carrying your subsequent babies since your abdomen will never regain its original strength *unless* you exercise. Most of the women we interviewed found that their waists had increased by one inch, give or take a few centimeters. This is probably due to the stretched abdominal muscles. This increase happens when you have your first child and, fortunately, not with succeeding children!

You may also be dismayed by the extra thickness of your hips, thighs, and fanny, or by "cellulite" or cottage-cheese thighs that you didn't have

Joanne had her baby just before the summer began. During the hot summer months that followed she found the early morning hours at the beach a perfect time to do her own exercise routine, designed to tighten abdominal muscles and regain her waistline.

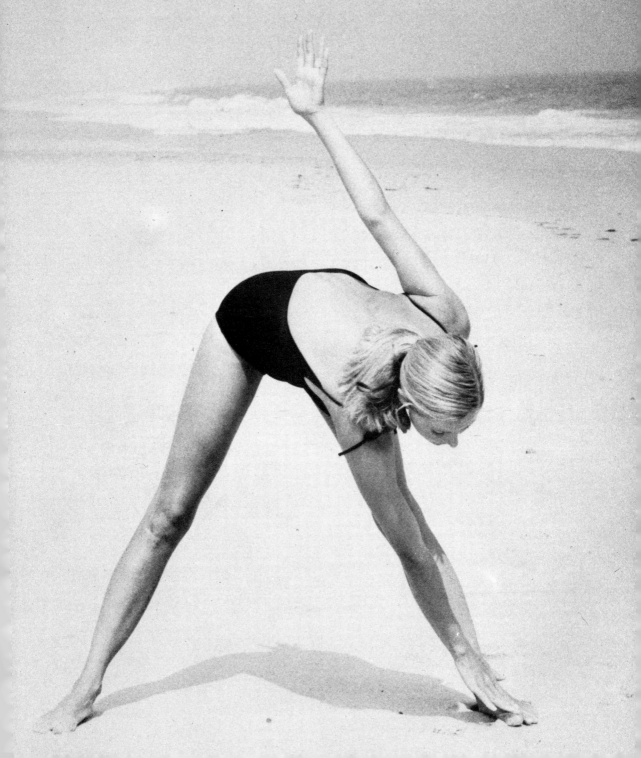

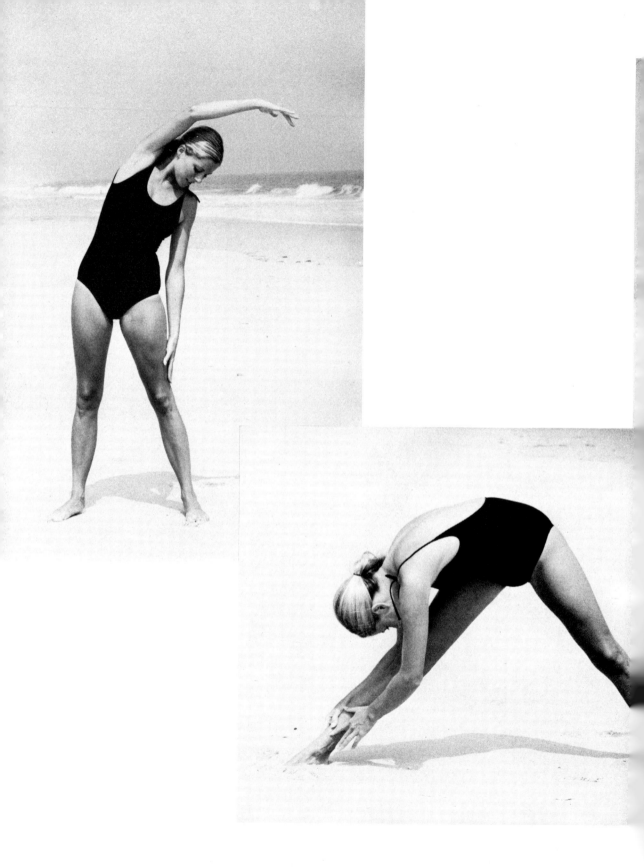

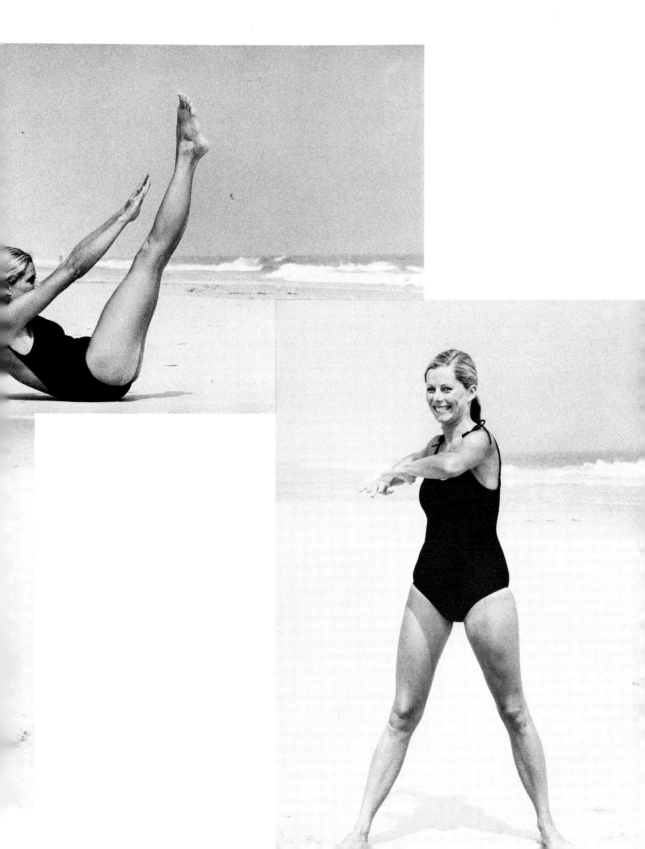

before. These are natural storage areas where fat is deposited during pregnancy, when progesterone may provide a stimulus to fat storage by resetting your internal "lipostat" or gauge. After pregnancy your body reverts to its normal fat regulation lipostat, and the fat from pregnancy is reabsorbed or lost.

Most authorities believe fat is stored in the second trimester by the greedy pregnant body to provide food for the fetus to live on, or to provide energy to be expended during lactation in the case of famine or other difficulty in obtaining food. Nature tries to assure your baby enough nutrients for survival, but since we do not live in a primitive culture, and have little trouble in obtaining food, this fat usually remains just that—fat.

This fat, however, is quickly lost if you are breast-feeding, watch your caloric intake, and continue a sensible exercise program (see pp. 225–40). If you're not nursing it may take months longer to lose even with careful diet and exercise. As long as your energy output exceeds your caloric intake, you will slowly lose this fat.

## VARICOSE VEINS

If you didn't have varicose veins before you were pregnant and did develop them during pregnancy, they may vanish completely within six months after delivery since the conditions that cause them have disappeared. As with hemorrhoids, if you had them before, they will probably recede to their original state or close to it.

"My baby is a year old now, Doctor," said a concerned mother. "And my varicose veins—which got worse during my pregnancy—are better than they were when I was carrying Jamie but are definitely worse than they were before I got pregnant." Her doctor reminded his patient that she was about two years older than when she got pregnant and that unfortunately, with age, varicose veins tend to worsen. Pregnancy definitely aggravates varicosities, but the veins may have degenerated from age even without the pregnancy.

Varicose veins can be treated. Unless you are in pain, try waiting a good nine months after birth and then consult a doctor specializing in peripheral vascular or cardiovascular medicine. At present there are two kinds of treatment for varicose veins. One method, probably the simpler, is called sclerotherapy. In this procedure, the varicosity is injected with a salt solution that eventually atrophies the abnormal vein and redirects the blood through healthy veins. The vein then "dies" and becomes colorless. A bruise may develop around the injected vein but in most cases this bruise soon disappears. The injection treatment is successful in about eighty-five percent of the cases and helps the look of your legs enormously.

The other method for dealing with serious varicose veins is stripping. This is an operation done under anesthesia in which the peripheral vascular surgeon pulls out the main vein and ties off the smaller attached veins. The deeper veins will take up their increased share of the work of returning the blood to the heart. The disadvantage of this operation is that scars show afterward. If you think either of these treatments is necessary, discuss the matter carefully with a medical specialist. (See pp. 106–107 for alternative or interim treatments.)

Many new mothers often attribute pains in their legs to varicose veins. "I suffered with aching legs for four months after delivery thinking it was varicose veins," said Ruth. "When I finally mentioned it to my OB she told me the aches were probably caused by two things: 1) the great strain put on the leg muscles during delivery, and 2) the uterus pressing on veins in the pelvis during pregnancy." Her doctor told her it takes some time for circulation to return to normal and recommended wearing support pantyhose. Ruth's problem subsided six months after the baby was born.

## NIGHT SWEATS, HOT FLASHES, AND PERSPIRATION

"I went through three nightgowns a night for two weeks," said Phyllis, a weary mother with a new baby. "My doctor never told me about the sweating and hot flashes you get after having a baby. I was really worried until I talked to another new mother and she was sweating through her nightgowns too."

Most new mothers experience nighttime sweating, hot flashes, and increased volume of urine—all of which takes anywhere from a week to four weeks to subside, as your estrogen level decreases and your body works night and day to rid itself of excess fluid or edema retained during pregnancy. The good news here is that many of the pounds you gained in pregnancy practically drip off now; the bad news is that waking up with wet bedclothes and limp hair, along with the baby's cries, does not add up to one's vision of beautiful motherhood. You can refresh yourself each morning with a shower. You may want to wash your hair each morning, too, while you are having these night sweats.

If you're perspiring excessively because of the stress involved in your new life, this sweat usually has an odor. Washing the underarm area with soap and applying a good antiperspirant or deodorant is essential. Keep a spray bottle of mineral water in your refrigerator and use it to refresh yourself whenever you are feeling hot or irritated. The mineral water also acts as a great setter for makeup.

## CAESAREAN SECTION

Once you get home you might find your Caesarean scar itching mercilessly. This is part of the healing process. Most women simply put up with it. Nurses we spoke to suggested applying cocoa butter to the area to minimize itching and keep the area supple. Avoid tight clothes and stay away from pantyhose if they irritate the area. Wear a slender garter belt with stockings instead.

## BREAST CARE—FOR NURSING MOTHERS

If you've decided to nurse you'll know most of the potential problems as well as the joys of breast-feeding your baby. But you may wonder about whether nursing will make your breasts sag, lose their shape, or get smaller. "My mother told me not to nurse so my breasts would look younger

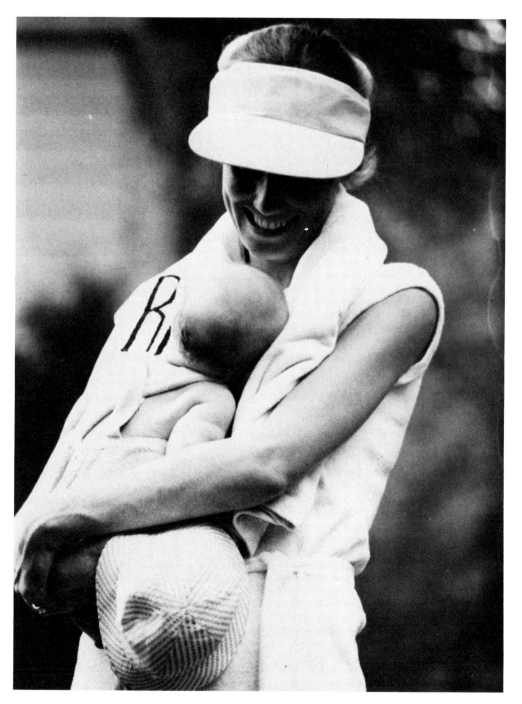

After nursing Michael, Liz is off to her tennis date. Contrary to what some women may think, exercise is fine during the breast-feeding period.

longer," Louise said to us. "Most of my friends told me to nurse. But that's because they were nursing too. Do you know when I made up my mind? When Kenny was brought to me for the first feeding. There was something so instinctual and natural about the way he followed with his nose and rooted around my breasts as I cradled him. I told them to hold the formula—I was going to try breast-feeding. Whatever might happen to my breasts was worth the magical feeling and the closeness of nursing."

Louise's doubts run through every woman's mind—especially those whose family, friends, and doctors don't encourage breast-feeding. If the look of your breasts is the prime determinant of whether you breast-feed or not, Louise's solution—follow your instincts—is the best. It is believed that pregnancy causes changes in the shape and skin of the breast, but there are no scientific data to show definitely that nursing causes further changes. Many mothers we talked to saw that their breasts were smaller and firmer after nursing. However, many nonnursing mothers also saw changes in their breasts. Every nurse, doctor, and mother we talked to said, "Go ahead and breast-feed."

Your breasts are even heavier now than during pregnancy because of the added weight of fluid and milk. Usually they require a bra one or two sizes larger. Blue veins often show through because of the increased blood supply. If you've had any cysts, lactating tends to exaggerate them. They fill with milk to become "galactocells." Although the possibility of developing breast cancer is less among women who have breast-fed, check your breasts for lumps throughout lactation (and throughout your life) for cancer can develop at any time. Report any lumps to your obstetrician immediately. Don't wait till you stop nursing. Your doctor can use ultrasound machines to test lumps without harming your milk.

These changes are mostly temporary. Those of us who take care of our breasts during pregnancy, nursing, and after, will look virtually the same after nursing. What should you do to make sure yours do?

- When you take a shower or bath, use your hands or washcloth to bathe the breasts and nipples. If your breasts are not sore or cracked, use a little soap and lots of warm water. Too much soap contributes to cracked nipples and causes you to lose all the beneficial oils on the areolas and nipples. Make sure you wipe all the soap off.

- Follow your bath with a pure lanolin cream—either hydrolanolin or special breast-care creams found in drugstores. Daub the cream on your areolas and sides of the nipples and the tips if you like. Most doctors feel it is not necessary to wash this off when you nurse your baby. For the rest of your breasts, apply a lanolin-rich moisturizer.
- Put on your nursing bra and open the flap to let the air soothe your nipples. Do this several times during the day unless this triggers your flow of milk—a response which may occur until your milk flow has been established.
- Make sure your bra is a supportive, though not too tight, cotton nursing bra. Cotton is especially important for the condition of your nipples. As we've said before, our advice is—wear your bra twenty-four hours a day! Your breasts will be heavier, several sizes larger, and in constant need of support in order to prevent sagging.
- Follow the general health rules outlined in other areas of this book. This is so important for a nursing mother and her baby that it can't be emphasized enough. Very simply, eat a good diet (pp. 241–57) and get enough rest, difficult though this may be. Nursing mothers need to follow these health rules more than nonnursing mothers to stay feeling and looking good.

## NURSING DISCOMFORTS

You can find information about the more serious problems of nursing—sore and cracked nipples, mastitis, etc.—in your favorite breast-feeding book. There is one minor problem of nursing, however, which tends to undercut the poise and confidence of the most sophisticated and chic nursing mother—leaking breasts. Leaking breasts can ruin clothes, bedding, and make you feel wet and sticky—day or night. They often accompany engorgement or continue after milk flow has been regulated. Leaking will diminish after a few weeks and probably stop after your third month of nursing. If you develop an eczema on the areola and breast from leaking milk or a baby who dribbles when she feeds, your doctor may suggest using hydrolanolin or a good skin emollient. If leaking breasts are troubling you try these suggestions:

- Try using soft disposable nursing pads which you can buy in a drug store. They can be used whenever you like, but change them often since the wet pads can irritate the skin and cause an odor. Use white cotton handkerchiefs to fit into your nursing bra at night.
- Many women find their bed sheets soaked with milk when they get up in the morning. Here's a solution: Take one of your baby's rubberized sheets and use it on your side of the bed, under your regular sheet. This will save your mattress from milk stains and odors..
- Are you waking up in the middle of the night with a wet chest, bra, and nightie and feeling just too tired to get out of bed and change? Keep one or two pretty cotton nursing nighties, two bras, and clean handkerchiefs at the foot of your bed to change into. Keep a few clean cotton balls and water at your bedside to swab off the leaking milk which can irritate your skin.

## BREAST CARE—FOR NONNURSING MOTHERS

Even if you have decided not to breast-feed your baby, it is just as important to coddle your post-pregnancy breasts as if you were. As the pregnancy hormones recede, your breasts diminish in size. You can gently moisturize and massage after a shower or bath with your favorite body moisturizer. Avoid moisturizing the tips of the nipples since they may be sensitive for the first few weeks.

## BREASTS AFTER BIRTH: CHANGES

Whether you have decided not to nurse or you have just weaned your baby, once your breasts have returned to their prepregnancy state (it takes about ten days after lactation has stopped for your lactation hormones to disappear) you may see some changes in their shape or the texture of the skin: stretch marks; flattened breasts; and crepiness in the skin texture. Pregnancy hormones and the prolonged stretching and stress on the muscles and skin during pregnancy is responsible for these changes. If your breasts have descended a little and you have never worn a bra before, you might start wearing one now and definitely wear one for the next pregnancy. Some of the light boneless bras are very natural and give you all the support you need.

Many women notice a flattening in the conical shape of their breasts. The loss of breast fat is most apparent in the top half of the breast—often making the breasts look less rounded. Some women who have large breasts welcome the loss of breast fat because as they get older, smaller breasts look less matronly.

If you gained a lot of weight during pregnancy and are now losing it, the skin on your breasts may look or feel a little crepey. This crepiness usually improves dramatically within six months. Keep your breasts moisturized regularly with a rich body cream.

Stretch marks on the breasts (see p. 113)—the result of less elastic skin, the added weight, and excess fluid of pregnancy retained in the breast—may be a problem for you. If you are bothered by them, plastic surgery is a final resort. One plastic surgeon we spoke to recommends an operation in which some of the skin on the breast is removed to flatten the grooves and streaks of stretch marks, making them less visible. The incision is made around the areola, skin is excised, and then the cut is stitched. A slight scar remains but is not very noticeable since it is close to the darkened skin of the areola. Other doctors recommend breast augmentation surgery, in which silicone implants are placed behind the breasts to fill out the flattened top of the breast, and tighten the grooved streaks of the stretch marks and the dry crepey skin.

Plastic surgery is a big undertaking, but many women are willing to try this radical resort to improve the look of their breasts. Think about it carefully and consult at least two plastic surgeons.

## OCCUPATIONAL HAZARDS OF BEING A MOTHER

In addition to the changes wrought by pregnancy and birth, motherhood can bring new stresses to your already overworked body. Joyce, a twenty-two-year-old mother, had very few physical complaints after she had her baby until one day her left forearm began to ache. She realized that a broken arm of her favorite nursing chair, an antique rocker, had caused her to support the baby at an awkward angle when she nursed. She changed chairs but her arm remained achy until she went to see a doctor and found she had developed tendonitis. With proper treatment, her arm healed within a few weeks.

This is just one of the physical occupational hazards of being a new mother. You often find yourself in such awkward positions as leaning over a tall crib or picking the baby up from a bed. Muscle strain is aggravated by the tension that accompanies caring for a tiny infant. You will have to relearn some of your moves in order to prevent backaches, stiff neck, shoulder pains, etc. Here are some common new situations you can handle with proper posture and new lifting techniques.

- When picking the baby up off the bed, follow the same techniques we described in Chapter IV, "Your Pregnant Body—Staying Healthy and Fit." Bend your knees, keep your back straight, and lift with your legs. If the baby is in the center of the bed, first draw the baby to the edge of the bed and then lift. When your baby gets older and is toddling around, lift him off the floor in the same manner.
- When putting your baby in the crib or taking him out, first let the side of the crib down. When your baby is very young, he can sleep with the side of the crib lowered halfway down.
- As Joyce discovered, nursing in awkward positions can cause muscle strain. Your back muscles may also tighten while you are nursing and/or snuggling your baby. Try to be conscious of your muscle reflexes. Make sure that when you nurse you have plenty of support. A pillow under your arm may help your arm reach a comfortable height.

- The shoulders and upper back are especially taxed when you carry your baby in a backpack or snuggly. See Exercise 12 in Chapter IV, "Your Pregnant Body—Staying Healthy and Fit."
- Correct posture is as important now as during pregnancy. As a tired new mother, you may get into bad habits of slumping, bowing your back, thrusting one hip out to carry the baby. Make a special effort to stand and sit straight. If one part of your body is out of line, the rest of your body has to work harder to compensate for it, leading to muscular tension and fatigue.

*All* these ills are most effectively dealt with when your body is in fighting trim—and the way to get it like that is with a good postpartum exercise program. You can start a serious exercise program three to six weeks postpartum *with* your doctor's okay. (Women who deliver by Caesarean section will probably have to wait longer.) Before three to six weeks your uterus is still involuting and your abdominal muscles are still shortening. Exercise during this time may cause bleeding. If you still have lochia, the postpartum vaginal discharge, and the color turns bright red, or you experience pain, stop exercising at once and report this to your doctor. After resting for a few days, ask your obstetrician when you can resume. Make sure you do just a few exercises very slowly at the beginning. If you feel well you can gradually increase the speed and number.

Although you may feel exhausted from taking care of your new baby, much of that tiredness may be due to boredom and anxiety. If you find it's difficult to leave the house, do your exercises at home with your baby cooing next to you or do them with another new mother and her baby. Choose aerobic exercise that increases your heart rate, thus stimulating your entire metabolism. The Royal Canadian Air Force exercises and the West Point Fitness exercises (both available in paperback books) are two excellent programs.

Set up a schedule with your babysitter so you can get out to exercise at least once or twice a week. If friends or relatives ask what you'd like as a birthday or Mother's Day gift, suggest a gift certificate to a nearby health

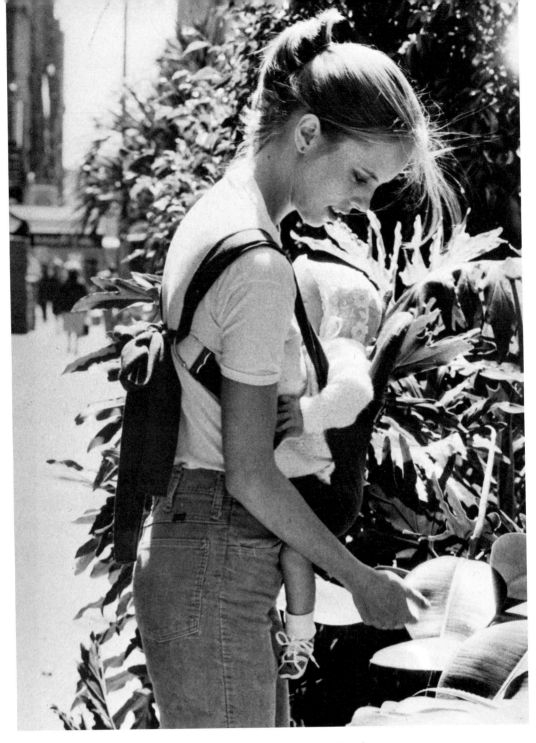

Carrying a baby in a pack can put extra strain on your back.
See exercises on pp. 228, 231, 235, and 236 for help.

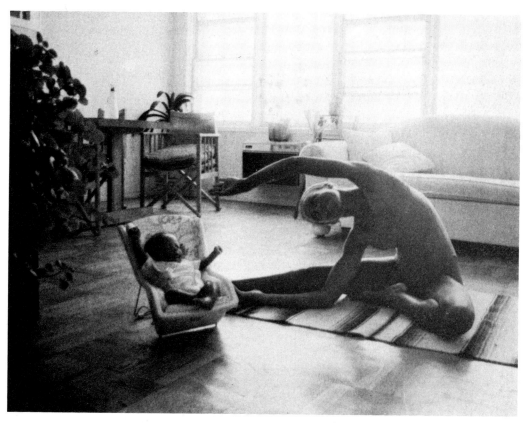

Soma enjoys watching Alva exercise and listening to her voice as she counts.

club. Make your exercise fun. Choose something you really like to do—ballet, volleyball, or horseback riding. In addition choose one sport, such as jogging, bicycling, or walking, that doesn't involve a special place, time, or equipment.

If all else fails (and you can afford it) go to a health spa for a week. Wendy, a friend of ours, went to a yoga-oriented ashram in the Caribbean, leaving her five-month-old baby with her mother and husband. At the ashram, she ate meals of fish, rice, and vegetables, exercised for four hours a day, swam, meditated, and rested. Until then, she'd been seven pounds overweight and feeling very flabby. When she came home she turned every head on the street.

## NO-NO ACTIVITIES AND EXERCISES FOR THE NEW MOTHER

Should you avoid any exercises and activities at first? When you come home from the hospital, don't run upstairs, or, for that matter, don't run anywhere. Walk slowly. If you jog or do other sports, wait till your first postpartum checkup and ask your obstetrician when you can resume these more vigorous exercises.

Don't drive a vehicle until you feel stronger—wait at least a week or two after you come home from the hospital. Don't do housework for the first week at least. Rest your body and treat yourself like a queen—you've been through a lot!

## EXERCISES FOR POSTPARTUM RECOVERY

On the next few pages is a program of exercises worked out by exercise expert Diana Simkin for postpartum recovery. These exercises emphasize strengthening certain areas such as the muscles in the legs and abdomen, and increasing flexibility and relieving tension in the shoulders and upper back.

Check with your obstetrician before doing these exercises—especially if you've had a Caesarean section. Some women are more tired than others and would rather wait two or three months after the baby is born. Gently ease yourself into a program when you feel ready. It is best to start within four months since after that your muscle tone will be harder to regain.

Before you begin these exercises, it is important to do some preliminary warm-up exercises that will gradually prepare your body for the more strenuous routine to come. Diana suggests doing prenatal exercises 1 (pelvic tilt), 2 (leg stretches), 3 (side knee rolls), and 7 (body circles). Remember to keep breathing regularly as you do these postpartum exercises.

The exercises on p. 239, for neck and shoulder relaxation, are ones which you can safely start immediately. (See Chapter VII, "Your Hospital Stay," for other early exercise suggestions.) Supplement the exercise program in the next few pages with a sport or more vigorous exercise class when you feel ready. By nine months postpartum you should be in top shape.

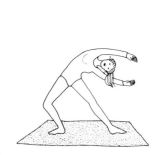
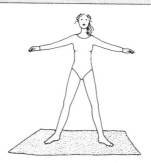
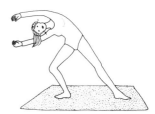

## 1. KNEE CHANGES

**Purpose: to strengthen the abdomen.**

Lie flat on the floor. Lifting head
and shoulders off the floor,
draw your right knee in toward
your body. (Be sure to hold
your leg below the kneecap,
not on it.) Lift your leg about six
inches off the floor. Inhale.

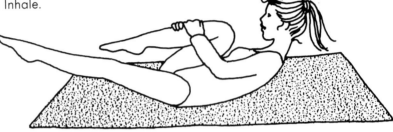

Exhale, flatten the abdomen,
and *slowly* change legs.
Alternate legs 10 times,
inhaling as you bring the knee
in to the body and exhaling
as you change legs.

## 2. LEG CROSSOVERS

**Purpose: to stretch and firm muscles throughout the waist, hips, and legs.**

Lie flat on the floor with your arms extended out to the sides just below shoulder height with palms down. Inhale and stretch your right leg up toward the ceiling.

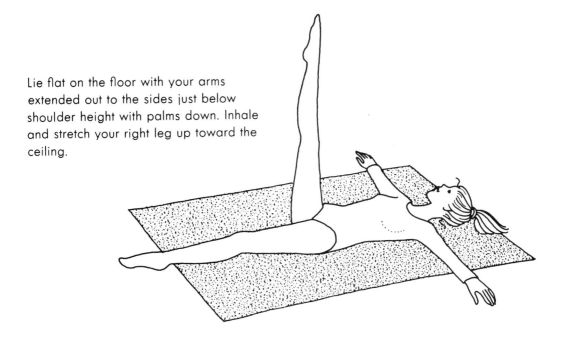

Exhale and cross your right leg over your left side to touch the floor. Try to keep your right hand in place.

Inhale and stretch the right leg back toward the ceiling.

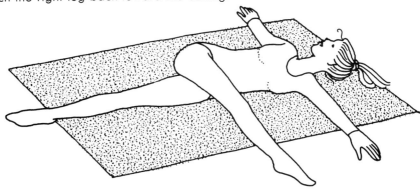

Exhale, slowly lowering your right leg back down to the floor. Repeat with your left leg, alternating 8 times.

## 3. THE WINDMILL

**Purpose: to strengthen and firm muscles in the waist, hips, legs, back, and abdomen.**

### Part 1

Lie on your back with your knees pulled in to your chest and your arms extended out to the sides with palms facing down.

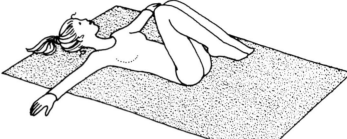

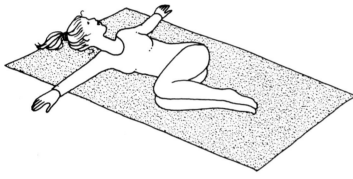

Roll your knees from side to side, making sure that your arms stay in place and that your back flattens to the floor each time you pass the center position. Roll 4 times to each side.

### Part 2

Begin as in Part 1, with your knees drawn up to your chest, arms extended. Roll your legs, with the knees still bent, to the right.

Then, slowly extend the legs along the floor so they are reaching for your right hand.

Bend the knees back in and roll to center. Repeat 3 times, alternating sides.

**Part 3**

Roll your knees to the right side and straighten your legs as in Part 2.

Slowly lift your left leg toward the ceiling.

Hold it there and lift your right leg up to meet it. Both legs are now pointed toward the ceiling.

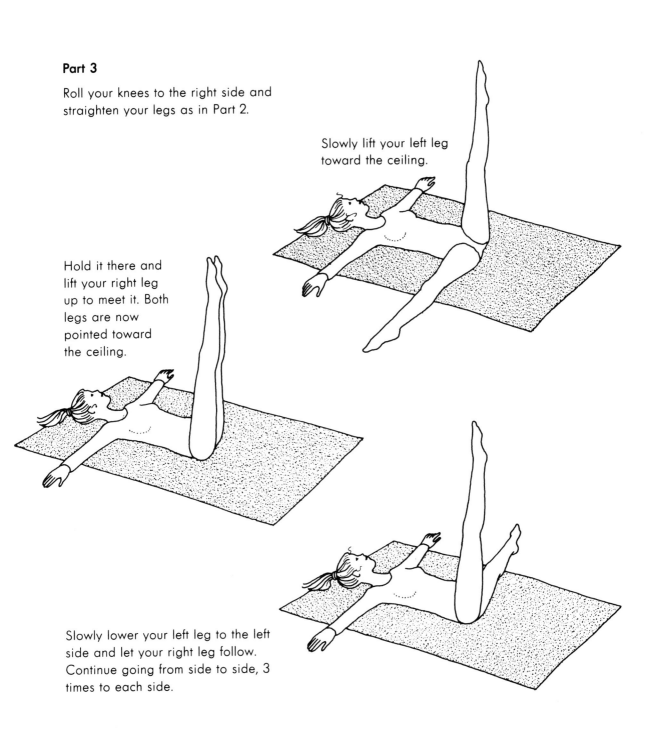

Slowly lower your left leg to the left side and let your right leg follow. Continue going from side to side, 3 times to each side.

## Part 4

*Don't try to do this one until you've mastered Parts 1, 2, and 3.*
*It should not be done earlier than four to six weeks postpartum.*

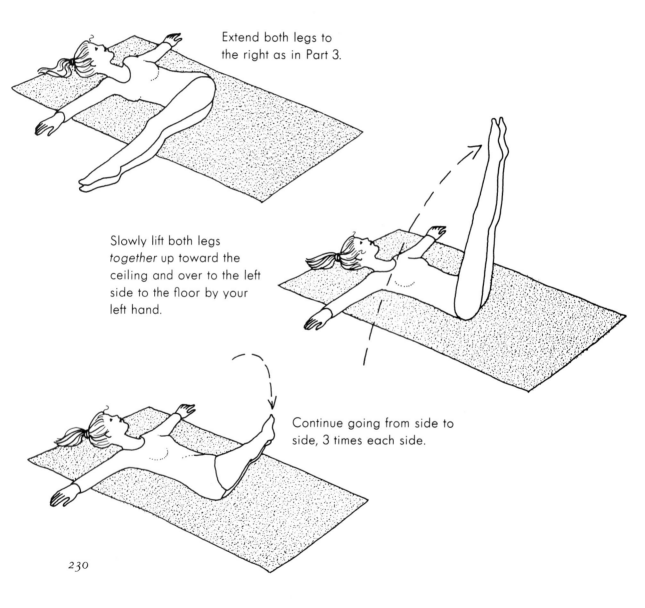

Extend both legs to the right as in Part 3.

Slowly lift both legs *together* up toward the ceiling and over to the left side to the floor by your left hand.

Continue going from side to side, 3 times each side.

## 4. PELVIC ROLL WITH LEG EXTENSIONS

**Purpose: to firm and strengthen muscles in the legs and back.**

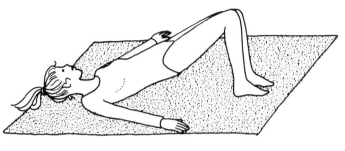

Lie down with your back flat against the floor and your knees bent. Roll the spine slowly into the air so that there is a straight line from your shoulders to your knees.

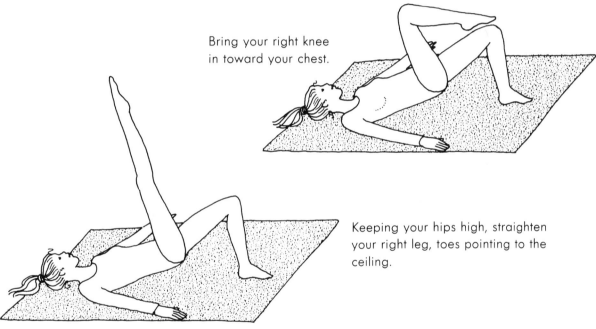

Bring your right knee in toward your chest.

Keeping your hips high, straighten your right leg, toes pointing to the ceiling.

Slowly lower the right leg, reaching toward the wall in front of you. Think of your leg going up and *out,* not down. Place the right foot back on the floor and repeat with your left leg. Roll your spine back to the floor. Repeat once more with each leg.

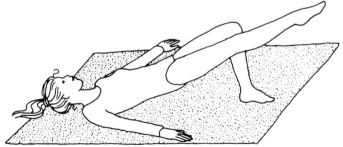

## 5. SIT-UPS

**Purpose: to firm the abdomen.**
**NOTE:** it is very important to do sit-ups slowly, using the abdominal muscles, not your shoulders and arms, to roll the back on and off the floor. In order to get a flat abdomen, you must keep it flat while you are working. Do not let your stomach bulge when you do sit-ups, even if this means only rolling halfway down to the floor. As your muscles get stronger, sit-ups will become easier to do, but it does take time. Remember, it's quality, not quantity, that counts.

Begin sitting with your knees bent and your spine straight. Let your fingers rest lightly on the floor by your sides.

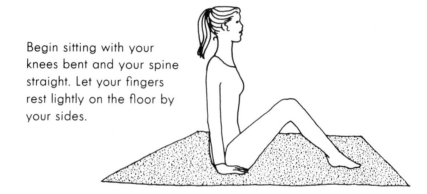

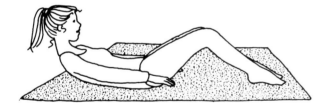

Slowly let the spine roll to the floor, feeling each part of the spine touch the floor separately.

Do not rest there. Immediately begin rolling slowly back up without using your arms or letting your feet fly off the floor. If you like, have someone hold your feet or place them under a bed or couch.

## 6. SHOULDER STAND

**Purpose:** to reverse the pull of gravity on all your internal organs and to stretch the back and legs.
**NOTE:** you may want to put a small pillow under your head and neck for comfort.

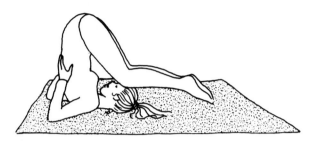

Lie on your back with your knees bent in to your chest. Roll your legs back over your head so that your knees rest by your ears. Place your hands on your back and relax into this position for about 15 to 30 seconds.

Slowly straighten your legs behind you. (If your feet don't touch the floor, don't worry about it—the stretch will come with time.)

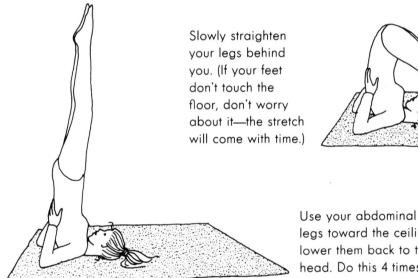

Use your abdominal muscles to raise your legs toward the ceiling and then slowly lower them back to the floor above your head. Do this 4 times.

Bend your knees so they rest by your ears and place your arms flat on the floor. Keep your knees bent in to your chest as you slowly roll back to the floor. Rest for a minute or so before proceeding to the next exercise.

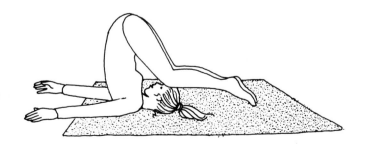

## 7. BODY CIRCLES WITH ARMS

**Purpose: to add stretch, tone, and flexibility throughout the waist and ribs.**

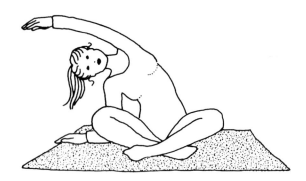

Sitting tailor fashion, bend to your right side. Place your right hand on the floor while stretching your left arm over your head.

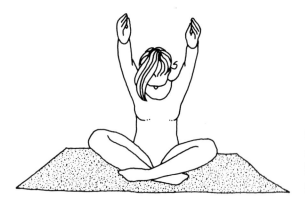

Reach both arms up and out in front of you. Stretch forward with a straight spine.

Bend to the left side, placing your left hand on the floor and stretching your right arm over your head. Roll up to center. Repeat 5 times to each side, reversing direction each time.

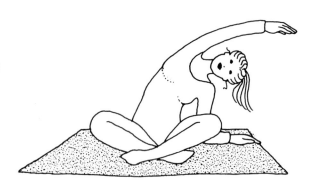

## 8. LEG LOWERING

**Purpose: to strengthen and firm the back and abdomen.**

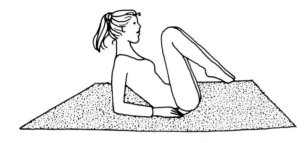

Sit on the floor and lean back onto your elbows. Bring your knees in to your chest.

Inhale and straighten your legs toward the ceiling.

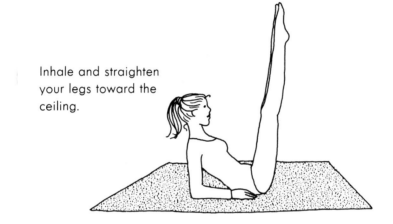

As you exhale, pull your abdomen flat and slowly lower your legs halfway to the floor. Try to keep your chest lifted, and your head and shoulders relaxed. Stop if you feel any pain in your back. This probably means that you are trying to lower your legs too far.

Inhale and bend your knees back in to your chest and up toward the ceiling. Repeat 5 to 6 times.

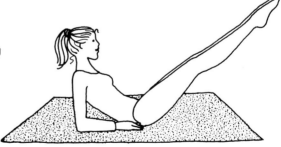

**9. MODIFIED GRAHAM STRETCH (adapted from a Martha Graham floor exercise)**

**Purpose: to strengthen and increase flexibility in the back.**

Sit up straight with the soles of your feet together and your hands resting on your ankles.

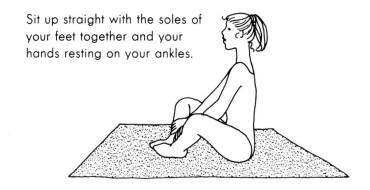

Drop your chin in toward your chest and roll your body forward.

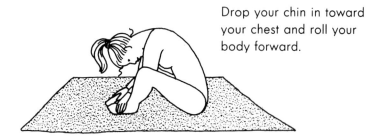

Slowly straighten your back so that your body is in one straight diagonal line. Check your position in the mirror if possible.

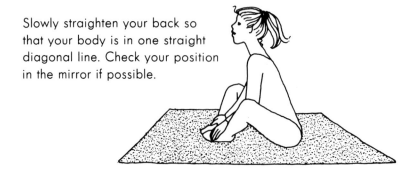

Lift your body back to center and begin again. Repeat 5 times.

## 10. FLAT BACK

**Purpose: to stretch the back and legs.**

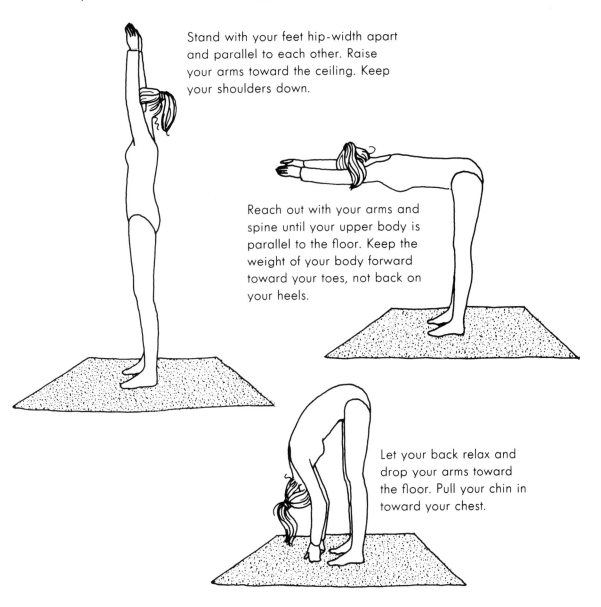

Stand with your feet hip-width apart and parallel to each other. Raise your arms toward the ceiling. Keep your shoulders down.

Reach out with your arms and spine until your upper body is parallel to the floor. Keep the weight of your body forward toward your toes, not back on your heels.

Let your back relax and drop your arms toward the floor. Pull your chin in toward your chest.

Slowly unroll your spine to a standing position. Repeat 4 times.

237

## 11. STANDING SIDE STRETCH

**Purpose: to stretch and tone the entire body.**

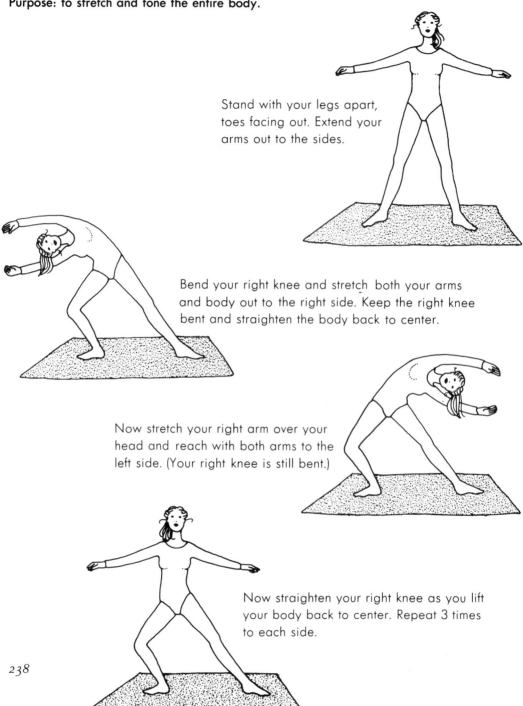

Stand with your legs apart, toes facing out. Extend your arms out to the sides.

Bend your right knee and stretch both your arms and body out to the right side. Keep the right knee bent and straighten the body back to center.

Now stretch your right arm over your head and reach with both arms to the left side. (Your right knee is still bent.)

Now straighten your right knee as you lift your body back to center. Repeat 3 times to each side.

238

## 12. ARM AND SHOULDER CIRCLES

**Purpose:** to relax the upper back and to ease tension in the neck and shoulders.

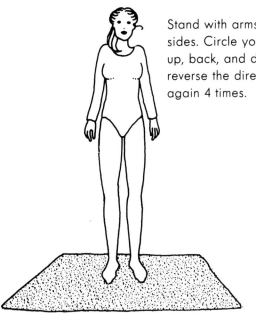

Stand with arms relaxed by your sides. Circle your shoulders forward, up, back, and down, 4 times. Then reverse the direction and circle again 4 times.

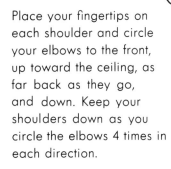

Place your fingertips on each shoulder and circle your elbows to the front, up toward the ceiling, as far back as they go, and down. Keep your shoulders down as you circle the elbows 4 times in each direction.

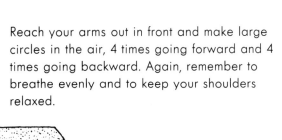

Reach your arms out in front and make large circles in the air, 4 times going forward and 4 times going backward. Again, remember to breathe evenly and to keep your shoulders relaxed.

239

## REVITALIZING YOUR POSTPARTUM BODY

It takes a lot of effort at this point to give your body all the special care it needs. However, if there is any time in your life when you should give your body maximum attention and pampering, it's now. Your recovery will be speedier and you'll feel better for it.

Within a few months, regular exercise is going to make a lot of difference in your figure and your energy level. We sympathize with all the women who have problems getting back to a regular exercise program—it's often very hard to pick up that thread. Remember that exercise is one activity that will bring about a marked difference in the way you look in a relatively short period. Exercise and body care, together with a safe weight-reduction diet, subject of our next chapter, are the most important ingredients of your postpartum health and beauty program.

# CHAPTER · IX ·
# *Diet and Nutrition for Your New Life*

"I WAS SO BUSY I could barely eat a thing when I got home from the hospital," said Jacqueline, a pretty French mother of one. "After eating heartily, and I mean heartily, for nine months, having no appetite was a strange sensation for me. And I was nursing Christophe—I needed nourishment. I think I was too tired. I lost twelve pounds in two weeks. I needed to lose them, but not so fast. I almost lost my milk. Next time I'm going to forget about the house, and concentrate on rest and eating well."

Many women welcome their lack of appetite when they first get home from the hospital. They feel heavy and want to drop the extra poundage as soon as possible. But *rapid* weight loss can leave you too tired to enjoy your new baby and new motherhood. Fatigue and weakness from improper nutrition can be rough on your body when you're tired from delivery and need strength to recover. If you are breast-feeding, you are twice as likely to get run down.

Some new mothers, however, overeat to compensate for the fatigue, anxiety, and boredom they may experience in their new role. Breast-feeding gives many mothers an excuse to eat heartily, so some even end up gaining weight! How can you keep postpartum weight down, or lose those troublesome pounds you gained in pregnancy, without depleting the energy reserves you need? What should you eat to keep you healthy and beautiful in this busy time? What special demands does nursing put on your body? This chapter tackles these problems.

## TIPS FOR THE MOTHER WHO HAS NO APPETITE

If you find that you are unable to eat well, especially during these first few weeks; if you've got circles under your eyes that no concealing cream can hide; if you find yourself racing around in the morning until—when you finally do sit down to eat your cereal, milk, and bananas—the milk has disappeared into the swelling corn flakes while the bananas have turned

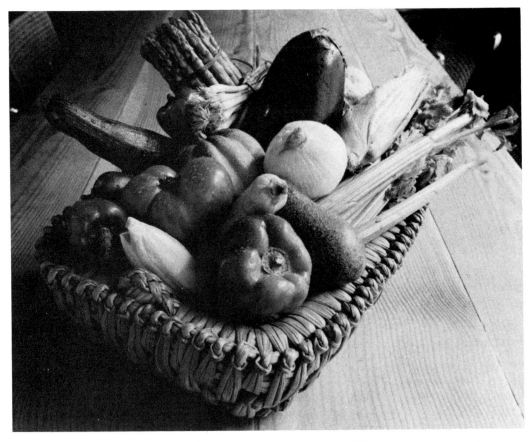

Think fresh and beautiful vegetables when planning menus. They're nutritious and can be prepared in lots of imaginative ways.

brown; what can you do? First, when you get up at six or seven to care for the baby, if you are at all hungry, ask your husband to get you some tea and toast. A small breakfast then, and another small meal after everyone's settled, will help you eat more. Help from the rest of the family now will set a precedent for group effort in the house, speeding the overall pace of your recovery.

After the baby's fed, your husband's off to work, and the other kids are off to school or otherwise taken care of, you can grab the morning paper and sit down to a second breakfast of warm oatmeal, milk, and honey, or poached eggs on whole wheat toast.

If you've had an early breakfast and are hungry for lunch by 11:30 A.M., by all means eat then. Don't worry about eating on schedule. Eat when your body tells you to. If you're not hungry at lunchtime, take a nap. This rest often improves your appetite. If you're very hungry at 3:00 or 4:00 P.M., eat your big meal then; at 5:00 or 6:00 P.M. it may be too hectic to sit down and enjoy a large meal.

As a matter of fact, dinner might be the least appetizing meal of all. Your nurse or your mother may advise you to let the baby cry a little while. "You just sit down and enjoy your dinner." As the baby's cries get louder and louder, your stomach gets tighter and tighter—until you throw your fork down and announce that you weren't hungry anyway.

We agree that it's virtually impossible to enjoy a meal while your precious baby is in the other room wailing, a sound other adults often seem impervious to. Try these suggestions:

- Prepare your dinner in the morning while the baby naps. Then heat it up at night when the chaos of the children's dinner is over. Don't plan to eat too late, however. You might lose your appetite and skip dinner altogether.
- Alternatively, you might want to eat your dinner early, perhaps right after you feed the baby. Later you can have a dessert with your husband while he eats his dinner.
- Try to relax before you sit down at the table. Have a glass of wine, chat with your husband, read an article.

## EASY NUTRITIOUS MEALS FOR THE NEW MOTHER

Whether you're nursing or not, whether you're trying to lose weight or keep up your strength, the key to culinary and personal success is the simple, quick, no-fuss meal. The faster and the easier the meal, the more time you'll have for yourself. Use all the modern conveniences available—pressure cookers, crock pots, food processors and blenders, toaster ovens, and so on. Swallow your snobbism about convenience foods, at least for now. Try some of these tricks:

### BREAKFASTS

- Frozen pancake batter poured from the container into a hot skillet.
- Cold cereal with fresh fruit and milk. Café au lait.
- Cold, leftover meat with toast, juice, and milk.
- Buttered English muffin with cheese. Grapefruit juice. Instant cocoa.
- Morning health drink

  Pour into blender—
  1 cup cold milk
  bananas, strawberries, peaches, or any other fresh fruit in season
  1 teaspoon powdered protein
  1 egg
  1 teaspoon honey or vanilla extract

  Blend till frothy.
  Pour into a tall glass. Have a piece of lightly buttered toast along with Morning health drink.

### LUNCHES

- Creamed soup from a can is easy and perfect for a breast-feeding mother when made with milk. Keep several types of crackers and cheeses on hand to have with the soup.
- Peanut butter is very nutritious. Spread on whole grain bread and add bananas and honey if you like. Peanut butter is also delicious with strawberry jam on toasted raisin bread.
- Cream cheese on date nut bread. Tea with milk.
- Plain yogurt with fresh fruit. Date nut cookies for dessert.

- Buy a barbecued chicken from the delicatessen for an easy lunch or dinner.
- Cut a fresh avocado in two. Fill with flaked canned tuna fish and dress it with a light vinaigrette.
- Spend a little more at the delicatessen section of your supermarket for sliced roast beef, baked ham, Swiss cheese, your favorite salami, etc. While you're walking the baby, pick up a loaf of still warm rye bread at your local bakery to have with cold cuts.
- Cheese, French bread, naturally carbonated water, and fresh fruit. Very continental!
- If friends or family want to visit you and the new baby, ask them to bring a lunch dish they can make at home or sandwiches from a nearby deli. Don't be shy! You need help as well as friendship.

DINNERS

- Roast a small plain turkey in the oven. Don't bother with stuffing or giblet gravy.
- Have linguine with canned white clam sauce. Serve with green salad and vinaigrette dressing from a bottle.
- Bake a 3-lb. ham from a can. For a delicious glaze, simply spoon a little honey on ham ½ hour before it's ready. Serve with marcaroni and cheese from a package mix.
- Douse a cut-up chicken with soy sauce and honey in a casserole dish and bake for 45 min.–1 hr. Discard soy sauce and honey after cooking. Serve with noodles and butter and frozen mixed Chinese vegetables.
- Buy the finer canned potatoes and sauté in butter and parsley.
- When you are cleaning raw vegetables for dinner, do enough to keep leftovers for snacks or to steam for lunch the next day. Or arrange canned drained vegetables such as sliced beets, carrots julienne, whole French string beans, artichokes in oil, and chick-peas on a platter. Pour vinaigrette dressing over vegetables.
- Broil any fish with fresh lemon juice and butter. Broil or grill hamburgers, lean meats, pork chops, chicken, etc.
- Have a canned dinner: canned ham, canned cranberry sauce, canned baby peas, canned creamed corn, canned fruit in its own juices for dessert.

## WHEN YOU GO BACK TO WORK

Working mothers have special problems—and not only because they have less time than they had before. Frustration or even guilt at not being able to spend more time with their babies can compound fatigue and weight loss or gain. As one new mother said, "Every area of my life is *so* disciplined now. I just can't seem to put restrictions on my appetite as well."

Many working mothers told a similar story. They freely admitted they used food to compensate for all the frustrations and complications of holding down a job and being a new mother. As time passes, you will work out your own ways to diet, but in the beginning try to keep fresh fruits and nuts in your office so you won't be tempted to run to the candy machine for a snack. Eat your big meal out at a restaurant (especially if a client pays!) at lunch time. You can then eat a light, nutritious dinner that doesn't take much preparation at home.

## NUTRITION FOR THE LACTATING MOTHER

One of the best reasons we've heard for breast-feeding your baby is how it makes you look and feel, in addition to what it does for the baby. Nursing is a terrific aid in recovering your figure: it helps involute the uterus and get your tummy back into shape, it burns off approximately 1,000 calories a day, and it releases nutrients such as calcium that are mysteriously stored during pregnancy and would otherwise remain as fat—fat that is especially difficult to lose. In order to keep up with your nursing metabolism, in fact, you have to be more attentive than ever to what you eat.

During pregnancy, your good eating habits are essential for the *baby's* health. During lactation, good nutrition is essential for *your* health. The baby of course is affected by the food and other substances you ingest, but not nearly to the degree that he is during pregnancy. Substances pass more readily through the placenta than through to breast milk. The milk production process draws directly on your body fat and, if your diet is inadequate, from other nutrient storages in your body.

How much should you eat? Estimates vary from 500 calories, as the government suggests, to 1,000 calories more than your *pre*-pregnancy diet. This is more than you require for pregnancy, but most nursing mothers develop an appetite that matches these caloric needs. Eating 1,000 calories beyond your prepregnancy diet is not necessarily excessive since you burn up approximately that much each day to provide a baby two months or older with his milk if this is the baby's sole nourishment. However, if you have a talent for gaining weight, you might opt for skimmed milk, broiled meats, poultry, and fish, and follow other sensible restrictions while providing yourself with the minimum daily requirements.

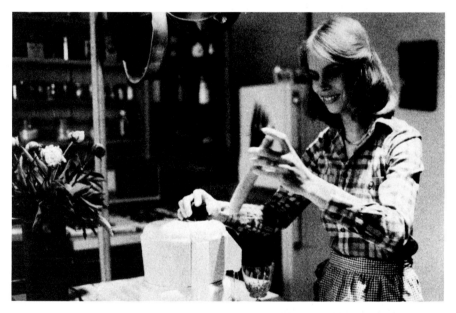

"LYNNE'S DAILY DIET" Lynne eats more now than when she was pregnant. "I'm so hungry all the time. It's a good thing my husband loves to cook." She often gets hungry when she's breast-feeding her baby and manages to hold her baby with one arm to nurse while eating a sandwich with the other. Lynne and her husband eat a mostly vegetarian diet (except for some fish and chicken occasionally), and have done so for years. Lynne's problem is the reverse of the one most of us have after having a baby—she has trouble keeping weight on. As a matter of fact, three days after her baby Alyson was born, Lynne did the enviable, if not practically impossible. She fit back into her prepregnancy jeans. Lynne drinks liquids all day long since she's been nursing. "My favorites are Perrier water and fruit juices, especially apple juice."

*Breakfast*
*Pancakes* ("Practically every morning my husband makes buttermilk pancakes. We have them with butter and honey.")

*Midmorning Snack*
*Milkshake with bananas.* One cup cold milk and one banana mixed in a blender.

*Lunch*
*Tuna salad sandwich on rye bread* and *fresh carrot juice.* Lynne makes juice in her own juicer.

*Afternoon Snack*
*Homemade oatmeal cookies with milk.* ("I like milk as a snack—I don't like it with my meals.") Or, *fresh fruit*—especially strawberries and watermelon.

*Dinner*
*Fish or pasta.* Lynne and her husband love Italian food, so they often make meatless lasagna or ravioli. Occasionally, she will make a *chicken dish* from a recipe handed down from her grandmother.

*Grandma's Chicken*

Cut up and sauté 2 medium onions in 2 tablespoons of butter in a large pot. Add 1 teaspoon paprika and lots of caraway seeds to butter and onion. Add 2 halved chicken breasts to pot and cold water to cover, plus 2 cubes chicken bouillon. Allow to simmer 30 to 40 minutes; then remove chicken and keep warm while you prepare sauce. Add 1 cup light cream to the liquid and thicken mixture slightly with 2 tablespoons flour mixed with ¼ cup water. Strain sauce to remove onions. Place chicken on a bed of rice and pour sauce over it.

*Watercress Salad*

To 1 bunch destemmed fresh watercress add either orange sections or apple slices. Toss with an oil and vinegar dressing. "We have this every night with our dinner. Watercress is cheaper than lettuce and high in iron."

*Bedtime Snack*
*Cheddar or Gouda cheese, with water biscuits or whole wheat crackers.*


WHEN CAN I DIET?

*Don't* diet rigorously until you wean your baby. You'll probably be dropping pounds quickly at this point anyhow, even if you are eating well. The government's Recommended Daily Allowance is 2,500 calories for a lactating woman who normally weighs about 128 pounds and is over 23 years old. If you hit a plateau during this period and cannot lose more weight, cut down by 200 calories. Try not to lose more than one or two pounds a week.

Although many breast-feeding books tell you to indulge yourself and dive into chicken kiev and raspberry trifles, this too is a mistake. If you gain weight now it may prove hard to shake later. Barbara, the mother of a two-year-old boy and a one-month-old girl, told us: "This time around I'm limiting myself to raw vegetables or raisins and nuts for snacks instead of blueberry pie. I eat plenty, but refuse to get into fattening foods again. I feel so much better after this baby."

The food groups listed in Chapter III give a good idea of what you should be eating during lactation. Simply add some nutritious foods to your daily intake. Try to eat high protein foods such as skim milk, eggs, cheese, and lean meat, balanced with cereals, whole-grain breads, fruits and vegetables. Avoid a lot of fats but give yourself enough calories each day to build and maintain your energy—something you need now even more than during pregnancy. For bodily functions and clear, healthy skin, you will need three quarts of fluid each day, since you lose fluid each time you breast-feed. Water, milk, fruit juices, tea, coffee, and beer (especially beer, which is made with B-complex-vitamin-rich brewer's yeast) all supply your fluid needs. Remember that tea and coffee are stimulants while alcohol is a depressant. Be temperate.

If your doctor approves, continue taking your pregnancy vitamins. If you feel tired or look sallow and run-down, you might also ask your doctor if you should take iron supplements. The course of pregnancy does deplete your system of iron and you've lost blood during birth. After a few weeks, however, you won't need iron supplements. Little iron is contained in breast milk so lactation does not put unusual demands on your body for this mineral.

You'll need to increase your calcium intake to compensate for the amount that goes into breast milk. Step up your milk intake to at least four glasses per day to keep your teeth healthy and your nails strong—or eat additional cheese, cottage cheese, yogurt, pudding, creams, etc.

## "I'M NOT BREAST-FEEDING—CAN I START MY DIET NOW?"

Many new mothers who aren't nursing are anxious to get back to their prepregnancy weight. But in the first six weeks your priority should be restoring your strength after the stress of birth. Since your body is still ridding itself of the fluids accumulated during pregnancy, you should be drinking plenty of fluids to replenish it. And you should be eating a well-balanced diet: high in protein, with some carbohydrates and fats, and perhaps a vitamin supplement to replace the vitamins and minerals that have been depleted by the stress of birth and mothering.

How long will it take to get your prepregnancy figure back? It could be six weeks or three months. One new mother reported, "It took my body a good six months to recover and regain its strength so that I could diet effectively." Other mothers we spoke to—especially older ones—felt that it took a year for them to feel well enough to diet and lose those extra pounds.

Eat well at first—about 2,000 calories per day depending on your height and size—and then gradually begin a weight loss program.

The substances that make you look and feel less than your best also have an adverse effect on your nursing baby. Although a smaller amount of drugs or unhealthy substances pass through your milk while breast-feeding than through your placenta during pregnancy, your nursing baby is still significantly affected. The following substances should be carefully regulated or avoided while breast-feeding.

— *Certain medications.* Check with your doctor before taking medications. An infant can be dangerously affected by certain drugs. Birth control pills are not advised for lactating women since the effects of these hormones on the baby's developing system is unknown.

— *Marijuana or other drugs.* Drugs do not sharpen parenting instincts. Marijuana is fat-soluble and readily transmitted to the baby and affects the baby's brain. It should not be used at all.

— *Tobacco.* Nicotine from smoking passes through breast to the baby. Cut down or out.

— *Alcohol.* Alcohol is a depressant and in addition to depriving you of energy, it passes through your milk and, in large amounts, can intoxicate your baby. Enjoy small amounts but don't overindulge.

— *Certain foods.* If you find your baby has gastric distress after you've eaten certain foods, avoid them while breast-feeding. Here are some common baby-tummy-upsetters: cabbage, asparagus, broccoli, eggplant, avocado, brussel sprouts, garlic, pickles, chocolate, pears, orange juice, and other citrus fruits. Too much coffee or tea can cause your baby to have an upset stomach, get excited easily, or sleep poorly.

— *PCBs, PBBs, DDT, or other contaminants.* Exposure to high concentrations of these substances may cause cancer or other medical problems for the baby. Therefore, women living in certain geographical areas around the country may have to sacrifice nursing in favor of formula. Ask your obstetrician for his advice. If you are at all worried about your exposure to these chemicals, write to the Environmental Defense Fund at the address given on p. 96. They can provide information on which areas in this country are the most severely affected.

## LOSING WEIGHT AFTER THE BABY IS BORN— WHY IT'S SO HARD, AND WHAT YOU CAN DO ABOUT IT

"I'm still eight pounds heavier than I was when I got pregnant," Judy told us when her son was eight months old. "My weight was always stable before. I just haven't been able to stick to a strict diet."

A year later Judy *was* able to diet and lose these extra pounds. Some women lose between 12 and 20 pounds by the time they come home from the hospital, and lose all their water weight by their six-week postpartum check-up. A minority even have trouble keeping weight *on* in this period. But by the third or fourth month after birth many women still find themselves 3-¾ to 22 pounds heavier than their prepregnancy weight, according to Dr. Maria Simonson of the Johns Hopkins Health and Weight Program. Some women can't lose this weight until six months after the birth, some don't until two years later, and some (shudder) never do. Inability to lose these extra pounds dominates the conversation whenever new mothers get together at exercise class, lunches, and playgrounds. We unhappily pat our round tummies, wear our size twelves instead of our tens, and never walk on the beach without a caftan covering our "little thigh problem."

## WHERE DOES YOUR EXTRA WEIGHT COME FROM?

There are physiological reasons that make it difficult for you to lose weight now that you're a mother. Dr. Steven Clarke, assistant professor of nutrition at Ohio State University says, "Due to hormones, women gain an average of ten pounds of fat during pregnancy. A lot of this fat is found in breast tissues and serves to prepare the body for breast-feeding. The rest of the fat deposits are found in the abdomen, legs, arms, and buttocks, and *where* they're deposited has a lot to do with your ethnic and genetic background. Some women gain in their hips and thighs, while others, usually thinner to begin with, gain in the abdomen during pregnancy. This fat is not easy to lose." Dr. Clarke says that nursing definitely makes you lose weight faster because the energy output in producing milk is extraordinarily high during lactation.

Another natural phenomenon makes trouble for many women trying to lose weight after their babies. This is *age*. As we have our babies and the years pass, our metabolism slows down and our energy decreases. The average woman puts on a pound a year from age twenty-five to fifty. After twenty-five we have to cut *down* on calories and *increase* on exercise to compensate. By the time you are thirty, your energy is decreased by three percent and continues to decrease as you get older.

ANXIETY, BOREDOM, AND FATIGUE. There are special, nonphysiological problems new mothers face in terms of weight loss: anxiety, boredom, and fatigue. No matter how "cool" you are, a new baby will cause you nervousness and anxiety of some kind. Many mothers respond to anxiety by overeating, because food is soothing and pleasurable. Further, although the baby is delightful, care for her can be repetitious and monotonous—especially when she is tiny. The kitchen is a great temptation and diversion when you get bored. And you're tired: what's a better way to fight four hours of sleep the night before than to eat high-energy snacks all day long? Carbohydrates give the fastest energy pickups, so we're usually drawn toward the buttered blueberry muffins or soda and corn chips. This is a trap that's hard to avoid. Many women confuse fatigue with hunger and eat when they really should be napping.

YOUR NEW LIFE CENTERS AROUND THE KITCHEN. Another problem you face is that life now revolves around feeding the baby. Women who used to skip meals, or ate out a lot, are now constantly preparing meals, snacking, and living life just outside their kitchens.

Dr. Sandra Haber, a psychologist who has treated hundreds of overweight patients, is always amazed at the number of previously slender women who gain weight during pregnancy and continue to gain because their new lives are spent so close to the kitchen. When the baby naps, the new mother gets company and reassurance from food. She prepares elaborate dinners to justify being home all day and to celebrate the one social event of the day with another adult, her husband. "The role of motherhood has been devalued," says Dr. Haber. "Preparing dinner and baking elaborate desserts can be the day's only creative outlet." Dr. Haber says new mothers buy more magazines. Women's magazines feature beautiful cakes on the covers, reports on the newest diets inside. Food is a way of relieving the unexpected frustrations of motherhood.

EXCUSES, EXCUSES. New mothers often consciously or unconsciously give excuses for being overweight. Carol Taney, a psychologist with the Connecticut school system, says that common excuses are: "In my new life the only thing that counts is the baby. I'm a mother now so it really doesn't matter how I look," or "I'll never be what I once was, so why try" ("If I don't try, I won't fail."), or "I want to have another baby so I'll just wait and lose all the extra weight at once," or "I'll do it when the baby gets older." Dr. Simonson has heard other excuses, such as "It's my glands." And she has noted the free-floating anxiety in new mothers—caused by insecurity and self-doubt—is sometimes projected onto their bodies, with weight gain as one manifestation.

You may not identify with any of these examples. But if you try to understand what is at the root of your weight problem, you'll have an easier time following your weight-loss program.

Being a new mother can help you work *toward* a slender shape—again or for the first time. The baby can help you rethink your eating habits. You *know* that nourishing your child is a tremendous responsibility and can't be handled carelessly. Your child will follow your eating habits. One friend said, "I finally learned I couldn't be a hypocrite any more. If I ate french fries and my one-year-old wanted some, I had to give them to him. I don't want *him* to eat french fries and I shouldn't eat them either."

Making baby food at home is gaining popularity. If you do so, you will be forced to watch what you have in the house to feed the little one. You can't grind up doughnuts and orange drink. You'll need to buy fresh, natural, unprocessed foods for the baby's nutrition. This also saves you money by shopping for only the best foods, which provide the most energy.

## "MOTHER" IS BEAUTIFUL

There's also the question of self-image. Becoming a mother does not absolve you from reaching and maintaining your fighting weight. As one woman put it, "No one wants to be a fat mama." You should try all the harder, since nothing is as attractive as an active and slender mother caring for her child. It's the ultimate beauty.

In setting up your weight-loss program, consult with your doctor first and then try to motivate yourself. Give yourself a date to reach a certain weight. Reward yourself with a professional photo session of you, your husband, and your baby. Or, buy a new dress for next season in your old size. Programs such as Weight Watchers, TOPS (Take Off Pounds Sensibly), Overeaters Anonymous, and behavior modification programs work wonders. They also give you a chance to get out of the house and see other people who have similar problems. Whatever you do, eat less and exercise more. Try these tips for losing weight and playing new mother:

- If you still can't fit into your prebaby clothes, pull them out and try them on to motivate yourself.
- Don't substitute food for sleep. You need both, but sleep never made anyone fat. Take a nap instead of snacking.
- Pay special attention to meal planning. Use a shopping list and don't fall prey to junk foods that are attractively packaged in supermarkets.
- Dr. Sandra Haber says that new mothers buy much more ice cream and "teething" snack foods such as pretzels, crackers, or cookies for the children. Before you had your children you may not have kept this food in the house. Many mothers get into the bad habit of giving their children one cookie and then eating one or two themselves. Remedy this situation by simply not keeping this food around. You'll do your children a favor by not giving them food as a reward. They won't grow up to treasure sweets and high caloric foods as tokens of their good behavior.
- Try not to spend any more time in the kitchen than is absolutely necessary. Have your afternoon tea in the living room instead of at the kitchen table next to the refrigerator.

- When you go into the kitchen, talk to yourself to inhibit the action of taking food and putting it into your mouth.
- If you must snack, keep a supply of nutritious low-calorie snacks on hand. (See pp. 91–92 for some ideas.) Make sure to take them along to the playground or beach so you won't be tempted to buy something less nutritious.
- When other mothers with new babies come over, serve tea or coffee with a fresh fruit bowl or fresh vegetables with a dip instead of baked goods.
- If eating out of boredom is your problem, try to have small projects on hand that you can pick up and work on easily. Why not take up needlepoint, a diary, sketching—or learn the guitar?
- Many new mothers get into the habit of watching TV while nursing and snacking at the same time. Snacking can quickly become part of this TV ritual. Change this habit now. If you find you can't give up your nibbling, at least switch from pretzels or cookies to celery, raw carrots, or hard cheese.
- Many mothers also get into the habit of eating what's left over on the children's plate. They've spent a lot of time preparing this food and figure they can't throw it out. Cover this food with plastic wrap and keep it in the refrigerator for tomorrow's lunch. Don't fool yourself by telling yourself it's going to go to waste if you don't eat it.
- Become aware of how much food you eat. If a diet calls for three ounces of meat, use a scale—not your eyes—to determine the weight. Also, be aware of how many calories are in each type of food you eat. Carry a small pocket calorie counter. Four pieces of apple pie can put an extra half-pound on you in one day.
- For your golden nights out on the town, order only one drink and a low-calorie entrée with plenty of vegetables and a salad if you like. If you love a rich dish with too many calories, order it and eat only half. Plan what you will eat before you sit down to a meal. Don't wait until you get to the restaurant.

Getting back into shape after you've had your baby is a challenge indeed—as is eating a nutritious and well-balanced diet during this hectic time. If you stick to fruits, yellow and green vegetables lightly cooked so they're still crisp and savory, milk and milk products (if you're lactating), lean, lean meats, fresh (uncontaminated!) fish, good breads and cereals, the world will be your oyster!

Weight loss will happen naturally for many, while the rest of us will have to try very hard to diet and keep up energy and good will on all fronts. It will be worth it—you'll be able to get into your old clothes or dress in some new ones.

# CHAPTER ·X·
# New-Mother Fashion

"I KEEP HOPING that next week I'll fit into my old pants and dresses," said Pam, a mother of a three-month-old, "But it just hasn't happened yet. I *hate* to go buy something in a size eleven when I used to be a size nine. It's like giving in. I don't want to acknowledge that I really am eight pounds overweight, my breasts are huge from nursing, and my figure's totally different."

Pam did get back to her size nine—but not until a year later. She was, as all new mothers are, very reluctant to accept the fact that her wardrobe might be out of kilter anywhere from two weeks to a year after she had her baby. Luckily, most of us resolve our figure and fashion problems within six months.

## FIGURE CHANGES MEAN FASHION CHANGES

Just as pregnancy is a time for special fashion consideration, so are the second nine months, especially for those nursing mothers who have a new big-busted look to deal with. Even if you've never nursed, or if you've weaned the baby and lost all your weight, your figure may not be the same.

*Opposite page:* Here's Joanne six weeks after the birth of her baby in a drawstring skirt, a cool T-shirt, and a long cotton jacket that slims her whole look. Joanne wore her drawstring skirt into her fifth month of pregnancy as well.

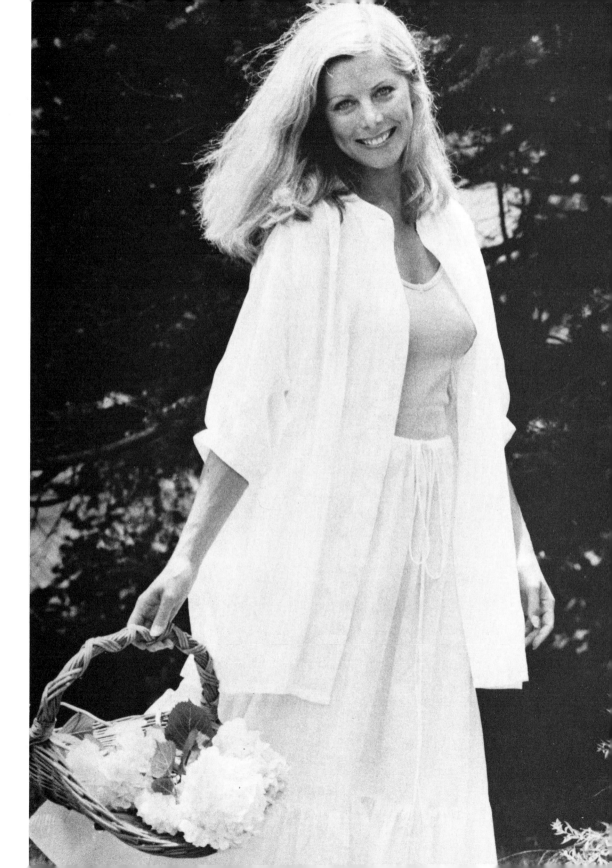

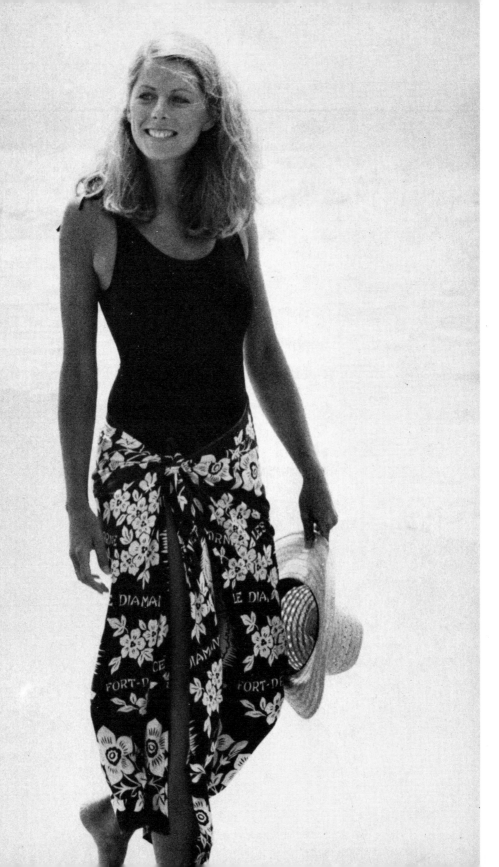

Your waist is larger, and your bust may be a different size. You may have some extra tummy or a little more padding in the fanny-thigh area that simply needs a lot of exercise. Or your hips may be *smaller* than they ever were.

Whatever figure changes you've experienced, your old clothes may not look the same. You will have to make some changes, either altering your clothes, adding accessories, or even buying new clothes. At different points in this nine month postpartum period, you will have to critically evaluate your wardrobe to outfit your still-changing body as sensibly and flatteringly as you can.

This chapter gives practical advice on how to dress during your first nine months postpartum. We offer tips on babyproofing your clothes and converting your maternity clothes. There are sections on shirts, pants, and the postpartum figure. Since breast-feeding presents a number of figure and fashion problems, we've included a full section about tops, bras, and nighties for the nursing mother.

## DEFENSIVE DRESSING—HOW TO MAKE YOUR CLOTHES BABYPROOF

Fashion problems you never dreamed of arise once you have your baby. "I just wasn't used to arriving at a party or at my in-laws with a rumpled skirt and baby spit-up on my blouse," said Linda, one of the mothers we interviewed. "If anyone stares, I usually tell them I'm bringing back the tie-dyed look." Boy babies may wet straight up in the air just as you're changing them on your lap in the car. The previous life of a well-dressed woman doesn't prepare her for the everyday accidents of being a new mother.

Leaking breasts can be embarrassing as well as hazardous. One beautiful friend we interviewed told us her most embarrassing moment in motherhood was when she and her distinguished writer husband hosted a famous senator at their summer house in Long Island. Her baby girl was then two months old. Our friend, with her new nursing breasts looking

*Opposite page:* If you have your baby near or during swimsuit time, you may feel too heavy to wear a bathing suit alone. This cotton sarong camouflages the common hip and thigh weight problem and looks exotic and lovely at the same time.

quite spectacular in her two-piece bathing suit, was serving hors d'oeuvres to guests on the beach. She leaned over to offer the senator crudités when she heard her baby crying. The sound triggered the let-down reflex which causes milk to flow, and her milk squirted right through her suit. The senator caught the two jets of milk square in the eye. He was surprised, but, as the father of three, very forgiving. Our friend's husband was so mortified he still pretends it didn't happen.

Fashion for a new mother is dressing for the unexpected. If you buy clothes during this nine-month postpartum period, seriously consider wash-and-wear fabrics. Or think about setting aside a little money each week for laundry, since you will have less time for this work anyway.

## CONVERTING YOUR MATERNITY CLOTHES TO POSTPARTUM FASHION

One of the biggest shocks after having a baby is finding out that you have to wear home what you wore to the hospital. Instead of slinking into the prepregnancy outfit you packed to make a fashionable hospital exit, you find that this outfit is too tight and uncomfortable. The shock continues as the weeks pass and you still don't look well in your prepregnancy clothes—at least the first six weeks postpartum, while your body is still involuting and your tummy and breasts are large.

You may be unhappy about having to resurrect your maternity clothes *after* you've had your baby, but you can give your pregnancy wardrobe a new look while you continue to make good use of it. Have your maternity pieces cleaned, pressed, and ironed, and add new accessories such as a natural leather belt or the high, high heels you've been longing to wear all these months. And try these turnabouts:

- All big pregnancy tops can be belted.
- Wear a sweater, vest, or small jacket over your old smocked maternity dress.

- When you've finished nursing, take in the seams of a pretty maternity dress.
- Wear a maternity dress as a tunic over the latest style pants. Belt or adorn with latest accessories.

## SKIRT DOS AND DON'TS

Skirts will pose the most frustrating problems of your wardrobe. The waist may be too tight, or your tummy may look bulgy in some. Your hips and thighs may be too large for your straighter skirts. Many of these problems disappear after your sixth week postpartum but some take longer. During this period certain skirts look better than others. Dark colors slim your look. Longer skirts are more flattering since shorter skirts tend to truncate your body. Soft cottons, wools, and better fabrics, in general, are more flattering than the cheaper stiff fabrics or clinging jerseys. During this bumpy time:

DON'T WEAR:

- Straight skirts, for obvious reasons.
- "A" line skirts in stiff fabrics. They're too severe for your figure at this time.
- Dirndl skirts. They have too much fabric at the waist and the extra bulk accentuates hips.
- Evening or "hostess" skirts gathered at the waistband. Many of us have these hanging in our closets. Keep them there until you've reached your goal weight and shape.
- Very full skirts. The extra fabric adds extra bulk.
- Unstitched pleated skirts, These are for only the *slimmest* among us. Bulging pleats are not pretty.

DO WEAR:

- A soft flow of fabric, which tends to forgive figure problems instead of highlighting them.

- Tiered skirts. They solve almost every waist-to-knee figure problem.
- Drawstring skirts. Pull them in as your body shrinks back to its original shape.
- Wrap skirts. Most will look fine, although those that don't "wrap" enough look terrible. A wrap skirt with a smooth apron panel is very slimming. Avoid folds coming from the waistband.
- A silk evening skirt with a front panel. It flatters your figure!
- Pleated skirts stitched from the waist to the hips. This type of skirt slims the hips and falls into a natural "A" line to flatter the body.

## PANTS FOR THE *ALMOST* PERFECT FIGURE

Here are some suggestions for the pants problem after you've had your baby but have not quite regained your figure.

- Drawstring pants.
- Oversized painter overalls.
- Maternity pants.
- Culottes in a silky, flowing fabric are great for evening wear. Short daytime culottes like Alva's on p. 267 are perfect for camouflaging heavy thighs.
- Buy a new pair of pants on sale in the next (gasp!) size. At least they'll fit and you'll look pretty during this period. You can always take them in after you lose weight.
- Pants with an elasticized waist worn with a shirt over them such as Alva's. She wears a pair of pants with a stretch waist and a Hawaiian print shirt for a comfortable at-home outfit.

## CLOTHES FOR THE NURSING MOTHER

"I've wanted big breasts all my life," said Marcia, a twenty-six-year-old mother. "Now that I have them, I hate them. I'm a 36D from nursing

*Opposite page: Suits are a great solution for women returning to work. They look smart and help conceal figure problems plaguing new mothers—especially if the skirt has stitched-down pleats.*

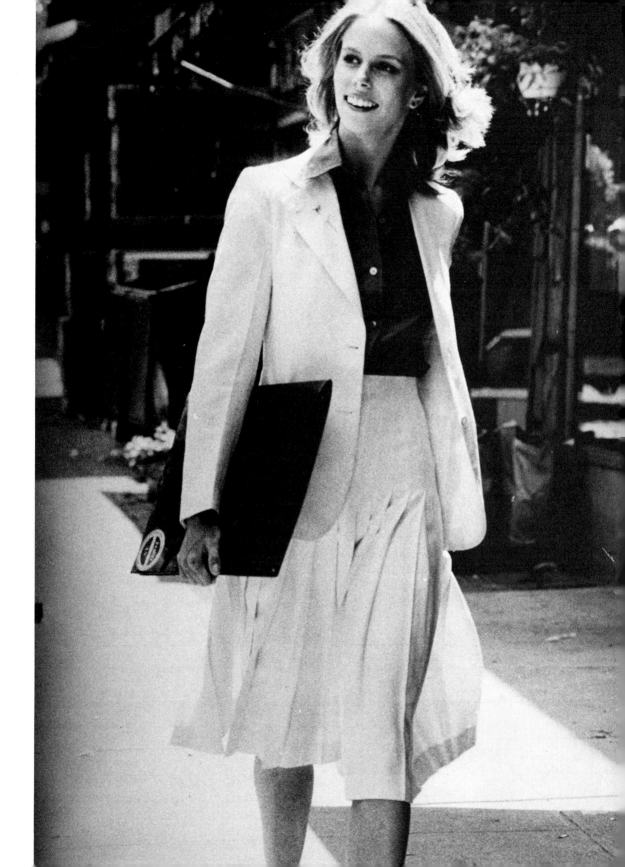

Danny and I'm bursting through all my shirts. I can't wear a lot of my prepregnancy dresses. On me big breasts just make me look heavier—not sexier."

Most women were surprised at the figure and fashion problems they experienced with their new breasts. Most of us think larger breasts will give us the hourglass figure male sex magazines feature, whereas in reality, larger breasts make clothes difficult to wear. As a matter of fact, the barer your outfit, the better you look. With your larger bust, bathing suits usually look fabulous while a blouse and skirt or suit often make you look dumpy. Once you wean the baby, you'll probably be happy to see your breasts return to their original size. Women who have always had large breasts and found them to be a fashion problem as well as an asset may lose some of the breast fat after pregnancy and nursing and they will look better in clothes.

Since you may have a big-bust problem for the first time in your life while you nurse, here are some fashion tips to improve your look in clothes.

NURSING FASHION DOS AND DON'TS.

- Don't wear shirts which pull at the bust line. This accentuates your larger bust and looks careless.
- Do wear clothes that hang straight from the shoulders.
- Don't define your waistline too much, contrasting the larger breasts with a small waistline. Wrap a belt loosely.
- Don't wear frilly blouses with lots of extra ruffles or fabric.
- Do wear darker colors that slenderize.
- Don't wear a gathered dress or top that hangs straight from the straps. A bust line that is fitted below the bust itself will give you a slimmer look.
- Do wear open blazers or jackets to cut the horizontal look of a big bust. (See Joanne at the beginning of the chapter.)
- Do wear bare tops that flatter a big bustline.
  (See Alva's top on p. 267.)

GREAT NURSING TOPS. Here are ideas for six tops that work well while you're nursing. You'll probably find a few of them hanging in your closet!

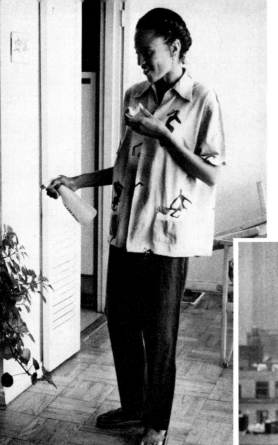

Alva's elasticized-waist pants and full shirt are comfortable, pretty, and flexible for her still-changing figure.

Alva plays up her new bustline (she's nursing) with a striped cotton halter. Culottes are great for hiding heavy thigh problems.

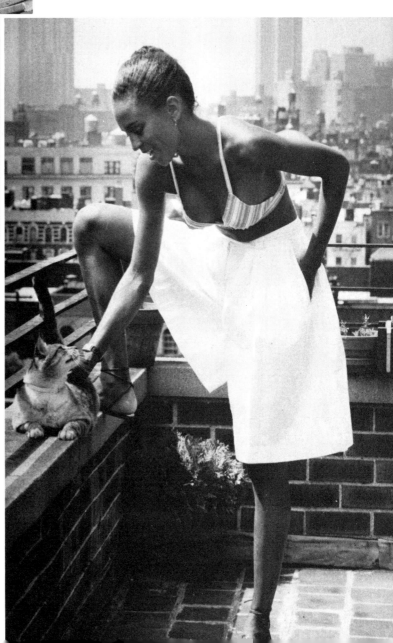

1. Big Greek cotton shirt with buttons down the front and belted is a natural.
2. Button-down man-tailored shirts. Add some accessories. (Unbutton the bottom buttons rather than the top ones if you want to be inconspicious.)
3. A soft T-shirt lifted from the bottom is easy to nurse in.
4. Off-the-shoulder peasant blouse, a style that has been worn for centuries. It's easy to lower the top and nurse.
5. Antique camisole tops unbutton easily and look pretty.
6. The smock top is probably best if you think you may have to nurse in public. If the top is blousy, it covers everything except the baby.

NURSING BRAS. "If someone invented the perfect nursing bra, they could retire for life," moaned the mother who was nursing her third child. "I've tried them all and not one fits well, opens easily, or holds up in the wash."

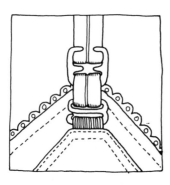

The hooks on these nursing bras are often difficult to undo at 4 A.M. They also catch in the dryer and break. Not our favorite.

Our research has not turned up the perfect nursing bra but since forms, sizes, and needs differ, perhaps there isn't any. Cotton fabric is recommended for comfort, but many women prefer a light synthetic.

You won't really know your size until your milk supply becomes steady. When you begin to cut down on the number of feedings, your breasts become smaller. You'll probably wear one cup size larger than your maternity bra.

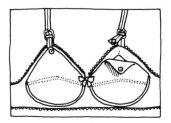

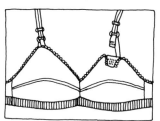

*Left:* Many nursing bras have Velcro tabs or snaps. These are often preferable to the nursing bras with hooks.

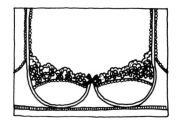

*Above right:* This lacy low-cut "French" bra is not only sexy but also suitable for nursing, and it has a good supporting underwire. *Below right:* This sheer bra is terrific because the fabric can be easily moved aside for nursing.

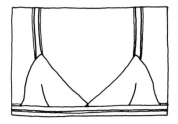

Look for bras in maternity shops or lingerie departments in larger stores. Ask a saleswoman for her help and advice when trying them on. Splurge on these bras once you find your favorite. The comfort is worth it. Wear a bra twenty-four hours a day while you're nursing to prevent sagging and to keep your breasts looking pretty.

NURSING NIGHTGOWNS. Ask for a nightgown designed for nursing as a baby gift. These nighties are life savers. They usually come in a cotton-and-polyester mix. They either button down the front, have slits for nursing, or pull down from the top. Choose the ones you like best. Invest in a few since they're fine for after you stop nursing too. Nursing nightgowns can be found in big department stores or at maternity shops.

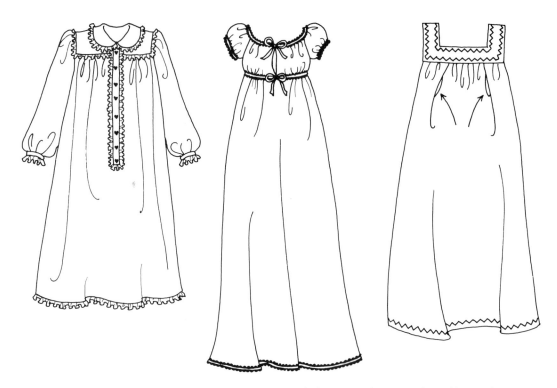

*Left:* A button-down nightie. *Center:* A gown with low-cut elasticized neckline, elastic under the bust, and small puff sleeves. *Right:* A nursing nightie with slits. These straps are wide enough to cover the nursing bra straps.

## NEW MOTHER FASHION

You can look as chic and up-to-date as ever after you have your baby. Your postpartum figure problems will be resolved and, for interim fashion problems, follow the suggestions here. Psychologically, now is one of the most important times for you to feel good and look pretty, so dress for new-mother success. Pay attention to detail—all buttons in place and no stains! You should be getting some of the admiring glances along with those given the baby.

# CHAPTER·XI·
# *Your Skin—*
# *Still Changing*

"GIVING BIRTH BECOMES YOU," said Aunt Mildred to Penny on her first visit to see the baby. Aunt Mildred was never free with compliments. "I'd almost say you look quite pretty."

Amazingly, the marathon of delivering a baby usually leaves you glowing—you're elated, everyone's congratulating you, and the thrill of having a baby and being the center of attention buoys your spirit and keeps you smiling. But often after a few weeks the enormous physical and emotional effort of giving birth, the hormonal changes, the nighttime feedings and interrupted sleep begin to get to you: a pasty face, oily skin, and circles under the eyes may be the result. Some skin problems caused by pregnancy may linger on, or only now become noticeable: stretch marks, skin discolorations, spider veins, acne, and a possible new skin change, crepey skin.

In this chapter we'll discuss how long it should take for these problems to go away or recede. For problems that are particularly severe or annoying, we've outlined steps you can take to attack them that you *couldn't* take while pregnant. (If you are nursing and strong medication is involved in the treatment, you will probably have to follow the rules of pregnancy and wait till you've stopped breast-feeding.)

For those who don't have specific skin problems, we're also including ways to make your skin look brighter and healthier. We've given you a

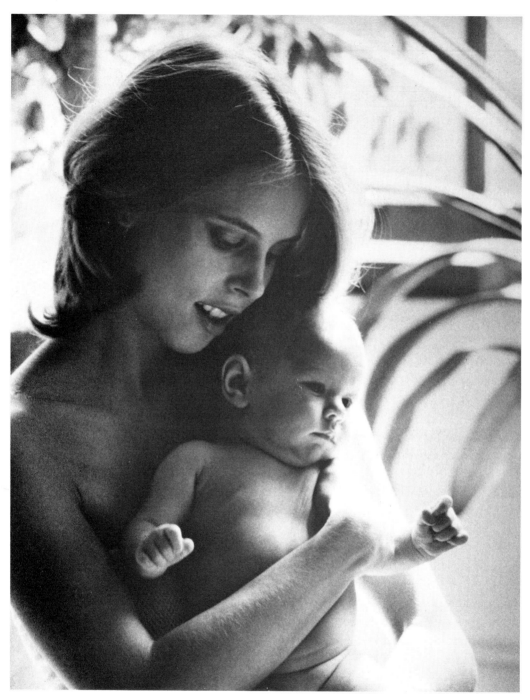

Lynne's skin care program has helped her skin look
as soft and glowing as her baby Alyson's.

new-mother beauty schedule and an easy five-minute makeup for daytime—with special tips to turn it into a dazzling evening look. There's no reason for the inner beauty you feel now not to show in your face.

## WHY YOUR SKIN IS STILL CHANGING

Whatever the changes you experienced during pregnancy, they are nothing like the tremendous hormonal upheaval your body goes through once you have your baby. The feto-placental hormone factory that, during pregnancy, had been producing one thousand times your normal amount of estrogen, is abruptly turned off when you deliver. Your body begins scrambling to return to its normal state in a mere six weeks—as contrasted to the nine months of pregnancy. Any skin problem arising during these six weeks postpartum is probably due to estrogen withdrawal. In addition, your skin may be affected by breast-feeding, since lactation further suppresses estrogen and speeds up your metabolism.

Remember that different bodies respond to pregnancy in different ways. One woman will have twins, develop no stretch marks, and have a flat abdomen within three months after delivery. Another will have a modest-sized baby and end up with a protruding tummy, stretch marks, and spider veins—because she is genetically more sensitive to the hormonal and other strains of pregnancy. This is not to say that "biology is destiny" and you can do nothing about problems caused by pregnancy. There's a lot you can do, from health and beauty routines and makeup to sophisticated plastic surgery. A dermatologist can painlessly zap a lingering spider vein or a plastic surgeon can get rid of flabby skin on your abdomen. Our cities and suburbs are full of well-trained doctors and beauty experts to help you look your best.

## ALL ABOUT LINGERING PREGNANCY-RELATED SKIN PROBLEMS

Soon after birth your big tummy is gone. For most of us, so are the skin problems we have developed during pregnancy. If chloasma, spider veins, or dry skin do linger on, they too will usually disappear in six weeks to nine months. But what do you do about them in the meantime? And how do you go about remedying them if they persist?

STRETCH MARKS. In our research and interviews we found many new mothers were extremely sensitive about stretch marks on their abdomen and elsewhere. Many—even the most defiantly "natural," let-it-all-happen women—experience grief or bewilderment over this change in their bodies. To some, the stretch marks mean the loss of youth. Others feel they are now flawed or less attractive. Some obstetricians we interviewed (especially male obstetricians) didn't seem sufficiently aware either of these feelings or of the possible remedies. But others were more sensitive. "Doctors shouldn't tell patients with bad stretch marks that they'll just have to live with them and wear one-piece bathing suits for the rest of their lives," said one. "It's cruel."

When we first started this book we were going to give stoic advice about stretch marks. "Grin and bear it." "Stretch marks are inevitable." "Stretch marks are the price of motherhood—and motherhood is well worth it." To some degree we still feel that way—but for women who are very disturbed by the look of these stretch marks, there *is* hope in plastic surgery (see below). But before deciding on such a course, *wait.* Remember when you first have your baby, your stretch marks will look reddish or brownish. Give them eight to twelve months to fade. They will look considerably better after this period. There are less radical techniques than plastic surgery for shrinking stretch marks, but their effect is limited.

*Tanning.* Tanning the stretch marks is recommended by some doctors. The ultraviolet rays may shrink these scars to make them less visible. However, some dermatologists warn that the sun can darken or lighten these marks so much that they become more obvious. "About half improve and half worsen with suntanning," says dermatologist Dr. Norman Orentreich. "If you are one of the unlucky ones whose stretch mark pigment darkens in the sun, there is a dermatological treatment to lighten the scar. If the scar doesn't tan in the sun, on the other hand, the patient should keep abdominal tanning to a minimum to prevent color contrast."

*Vitamin E.* Some women we've interviewed swear that vitamin E heals stretch marks and other scars effectively. Says Nima, mother of a six-month-old, "Simply break one capsule of vitamin E and rub it over your scar. Do this twice a day and you will see a change in three months." Many scientists disagree, reporting that vitamin E has no beneficial effect when applied topically to scars. Since vitamin E does no harm, it may be worth trying. Make up your own mind.

*Exercise.* Loose, flabby skin allows the stretch marks to become compressed, catching the light and therefore becoming more obvious. A firm, taut abdomen (see exercises on pp. 226, 228–30, 232, and 235) means that there is less flab for the stretch mark scars to sink into. The stretch marks are then not as noticeable.

There are some remedies for stretch marks that may *seem* helpful, but are ineffective and possibly harmful. *Don't* try the following:

*Makeup.* Even theatrical makeup or special covering creams do not work very well to cover stretch marks, and they may make the scars look worse. Stretch mark scars are usually depressed, so there is no flat surface on which to apply the makeup. And, when you're seated, the folds of the abdomen rub together and remove the makeup.

*Dermabrasion.* Although a few doctors use this method, the results, according to Dr. Orentreich, are scars worse than those you started with. "Abrasion surgery works very well when you have thick, normal skin, especially on the face. Dermabrasion *off* the face is a problem, and on very thin tissue, such as stretch mark scars, it can be a disaster."

*Plastic Surgery as a Last Resort.* Our last suggestion—and a last resort—is plastic surgery. This operation, called an "abdominoplasty" or "abdominal lipectomy," removes the part of the abdominal skin that bears the stretch marks. A large incision is made side to side on the upper level of the pubic bone (much like the bikini cut for the Caesarean section delivery) and another incision is made around the belly button. The skin is actually lifted off the abdomen, and the abdominal muscles, which may have been torn and stretched out during pregnancy, are tightened by sutures and folded into the abdomen so they won't pouch out. The old skin with stretch marks from this area is excised and the skin from the rib cage to the waist is then stretched down over the lower abdomen and sewn to the skin above the pubic bone. A new hole for the belly button is cut and sutured. The operation is performed under anesthesia in a hospital. It requires a stay of approximately five days and a \$2500 to \$3500 fee plus hospital expenses. According to doctors who have performed the operation, in three weeks you should be back to your normal activities.

Obviously this kind of treatment won't be appropriate for everyone. According to Dr. Robert Schwager, a New York plastic surgeon, the ideal candidate for the operation is a woman who has 1) loose flabby skin, 2) lower abdominal stretch marks, and 3) relaxed stomach muscles; the abdominoplasty is usually effective in treating these three problems. But several words of caution are necessary. Before you decide to have plastic surgery, be aware of the fact that if you have any more children, another pregnancy might cause more stretch marks. You should also be realistic about the results—one scar is traded for another and sometimes the results are not up to your expectations. And finally, remember that plastic surgery is a big undertaking, both psychologically and financially. Although complications are rare, be prepared for them. Most important, discuss *all* aspects of the operation with your doctor—who should be certified by the American Board of Plastic Surgery. Then get at least one other opinion.

CHLOASMA—MASK OF PREGNANCY. Although most cases of chloasma fade away in three months to a year, breast-feeding may prolong the effects—so if you're nursing, you'll have to wait until two or three months after weaning to see if your chloasma changes. In the meantime, try the makeup tips on pp. 15–16 to even your coloring. Stay out of the sun: exposure to the sun can prolong and deepen chloasma even after you give birth.

If you do decide that your hyperpigmentation is not going away and you want to seek treatment, shop around for a good dermatologist who is experienced in handling problems of chloasma. Ask friends, other doctors, and the hospital for advice. The doctor's skill is of utmost significance. As Dr. Orentreich explains, "It's just like art—a paintbrush in the hands of two different people can produce either something beautiful or something that is unacceptable to the eye. Judgment and knowledge, how much chemical to apply, how frequently, how much to neutralize, is an art and science." There are, in fact, several treatments for this problem:

*Peeling or Exfoliation.* With this, the most popular method of treatment, mild astringents and chemical agents are applied to the chloasma to "burn" the top layer of the skin. This then peels off, allowing the skin underneath to show through. This procedure isn't foolproof: the results do not satisfy many women. This and other treatments listed below may cause temporary unsightly results requiring the patient to stay out of view while they are treated.

*Bleaching Preparations.* With this method, the dermatologist actually bleaches the hyperpigmentation so it matches the rest of your skin. One dermatologist warns that the prognosis for change is guarded. One in six patients' skin will react allergically to the strong chemicals in the bleaching cream or lotion.

*Exfoliation and Bleaching.* Some doctors combine the two methods above and get good results; the risks and benefits are as described above.

*Dermabrasion.* As a last resort, some dermatologists will try abrading or planing the top layer of the skin with a dermabrasion machine. This method is successful in approximately thirty percent of the cases, and is very drastic. It is painful and can leave permanent scars if done improperly.

*Cryotherapy.* This is another last resort and again is successful only about thirty percent of the time. In cryotherapy, liquid nitrogen is sprayed or applied on the pigmented area. If too much is used, depigmentation occurs. Because of the unpredictability of the outcome, cryotherapy on chloasma is rarely indicated.

Whatever you do, make sure you don't treat chloasma yourself. Remember most cases of chloasma don't require any special attention; they disappear by themselves. As Dr. Charles DeFeo, dermatologist at Lenox Hill Hospital, observes, "I've never seen a sixty-year-old woman with chloasma. This is proof that it does go away."

LINEA NIGRA. Although one obstetrician we interviewed believes the linea nigra—the brown pigmented line resulting from pregnancy running from the top of the pubic bone to the navel—never completely fades away, a check with our mother friends found the opposite to be true. Most said the line had totally disappeared in six months to a year after they had their babies.

Dermatologists and obstetricians we talked to reported they had never received a request to remove a persistent linea nigra. "Women just accept it," said one. The recommendation is to leave this line alone. Don't try to treat it yourself with bleaching creams or peeling agents. What you can do is tighten your tummy with exercise—this helps the whole look of your abdomen.

SPIDER VEINS—SPIDER ANGIOMAS OR SPIDER NEVAE. Spider veins should clear up anytime from two weeks to six months after giving birth. If your spider veins persist for longer than six months, you might talk to your dermatologist about having them removed by electrolysis, a process in which the doctor destroys the vein by injecting it with a small electric needle. There are two drawbacks to this treatment: the needle may leave a small hole where the vein used to be, and the spiders will probably recur on the same sites in the next pregnancy. You may therefore want to have all your children before trying this treatment. Meanwhile follow the suggestions on p. 19 for covering these veins.

ACNE. Pregnancy-related acne typically clears up quickly after delivery but some cases do not give up so easily. Fortunately, there are many ways to attack it now that you are not pregnant. If you are nursing, it is better to wait until after you've weaned to take any oral medication, but you can apply topical antibiotics such as tetracycline and erythromycin to the skin. Topical vitamins also work for many women. Your dermatologist may prescribe a medicated complexion soap to use twice a day. Cover-up products are helpful to both the nursing and nonnursing mother with acne. You might ask your dermatologist for a medicated foundation. However, use makeup sparingly so your skin has a chance to heal.

Once you stop nursing, your dermatologist might prescribe an oral antibiotic such as tetracycline (though she should warn you about the possible side effects). Steroid hormones are also gaining popularity as an acne treatment. If you begin taking birth control pills after having the baby, they will add estrogen in controlled amounts to your system, which also may help control acne.

DRY SKIN—OILY SKIN. "Why did I have to get oily skin now?" new mother Rebecca lamented. "At twenty-five, it's not like I am a teenager. Do you think the baby caused it?"

Skin can become spontaneously oily or dry during pregnancy (see pp. 21–25) or after. Scientists don't really understand why but assume that the hormonal upheaval of pregnancy and the postpartum period must have something to do with it. Stress, fatigue, diet, and the rigors of a tiring schedule may also contribute. Pregnancy-related oiliness or dryness will probably reverse itself a few months after delivery (or weaning, if you are a nursing mother). While you have a problem, you can treat yourself with one of the skin care routines on pp. 21–27. Your skin will look brighter and clearer once you start caring for it with regularity.

CREPEY SKIN—A NEW PROBLEM. After the baby is born and you start losing weight, you may notice a new problem caused by the added weight and bulk of pregnancy—crepey skin. You may see anything from a slight crepiness to a large expanse of dry, sagging skin somewhere on your body—most commonly on the breasts and abdomen, but also on the upper legs, arms, or any area where you gained weight and retained fluid while you were pregnant. (Breast-feeding mothers often don't see the full effects until after they've stopped nursing.)

What has happened is that the collagen in our body tissues has given out under the stress of additional hormones, fluid, and fat. And of course the baby has stretched the skin enormously. What can you do about it?

- Use a loofah or a similar synthetic sponge on the affected areas while you bathe, always rubbing gently on your breasts. This gentle friction will slough off the top layer of dry, flaky skin and allow the smooth, clear new skin to show through.
- Moisturize with an enriching body lotion every morning, every night, and right after bathing, always applying with a gentle upward motion.
- Every day, do the abdominal exercises described on pp. 226, 228–30, 232, and 235. A tighter abdomen will give your skin less chance to fold and look crepey. For crepey skin on the breasts, do the pectoral muscle exercise on p. 239.
- The crepey flesh on the breasts, abdomen, thighs, and buttocks can be remedied to some degree by plastic surgery, although this will leave a scar. Talk to a good plastic surgeon about this operation.

## YOUR NEW-MOTHER BEAUTY PROGRAM

"I saw Ellen in the park a month after she had Teddy," reported Kay. "I couldn't believe my eyes. Her skin was glowing, she wore makeup, and everything about her looked fresh and neat. I really admired Ellen for pulling herself together like that. I know how difficult it was after I had my baby. I felt my skin aged twenty years—I looked so washed out."

Your friends' reaction to your appearance and composure after you deliver is very important—to both you and them. People will be visiting you and assessing how you are handling the great upheaval of having a baby. It's up to you not to let the demands of your new life take a toll on your face. A beauty routine may seem like the last priority when there are dishes to do and beds to make, but remember that a new mother who *looks* less than her best often *feels* less than her best. What you lack in inner energy can be made up for by some wonderful skin-energizing methods and machines, some old and some brand-new. Take advantage of facial sauna machines, skin cleansing machines, cleansing grains, astringents, toners, and masks. They all work to energize and clean your skin by removing the layer of dead skin cells that build up on your face. They're great pick-me-ups and will leave your skin feeling tight and tingly.

In addition, try these techniques to get back the glow of health:

- Use a moderate amount of makeup when you are fatigued. More makeup doesn't correct less sleep—and may make you look worse.
- For daytime, try a tinted moisturizer instead of a foundation to pick up the color in your face.
- If your pale skin is on the sallow side use a foundation with a pink tint all over your face, blending well into your neck. This will correct the yellow in your skin and give you a healthier look.
- A rose or pink gel stick blusher will do wonders for a pale, drawn face. Dot on and blend in the color at the temples, the cheeks, the tip of your nose, and chin—places where the sun would naturally highlight your skin. This will give you a "just off the ski slope" rather than a "just out of the hospital" look.
- Another instant beautifier is a bronzer. Your husband might want to try it too!
- If you've never been an exercise fan before, you might be inspired now when your prepregnancy figure and pretty skin are the rewards. Exercise improves circulation and gives you the least expensive and most natural skin glow of all.

How do you make time to care for *you* when most of your day is devoted to caring for your baby? Here is a schedule of beauty routines that revolves around the imaginary perfect new baby. Use it as a sample to set up your own schedule that provides time for yourself during the day and time for you and your husband at night. As time goes on, you'll be able to expand your activities and these beauty tricks will become second nature. If you're a working mother, when you return to your job, you can use the pre- and post-job-hour tips. Makeup can be refreshed at work.

| | |
|---|---|
| 6:00 A.M. | Baby awakens. Feed and change her. Cleanse face with cotton moistened with an astringent or toner. Rinse with tepid water. Apply moisturizer. Use a clear lip gloss. |
| 7:00 A.M. | Breakfast—make it a good one, you'll need it! Shower or bathe to start the day off fresh. Take the time to pour a capful of bath oil into the tub. Use this bath time to push back cuticles and rub rough spots on heels and elbows with a pumice stone. Rub in a good lubricating lotion on still-damp skin. Pull hair up with pretty ribbons or combs. |
| 10:00 A.M. | Feed baby and put her in for (hopefully!) a nap. You've already been up for four hours and you feel like it's dinner time. During the first few weeks try to nap along with the baby. Rest and sleep are the best skin-improvers at this stage. This is a perfect time to use a rich eye cream. |
| 11:30 A.M. | Apply daytime makeup now. Your baby may be the only one who sees you, but you'll feel one hundred times better! |
| 12:00 P.M. | Eat a lunch high in protein. Include a green salad with oil and vinegar dressing and fresh fruit. Don't forget a glass of milk if you're nursing. |
| 2:00 P.M. | Feed baby. |
| 3:00 P.M. | Relaxation time. Sink into a comfortable chair. Close your eyes and put cucumber slices on the lids—it makes them feel cool and refreshed. Or use |

|  |  |
|---|---|
| | this quiet time to read a chapter in one of your baby-care books. |
| 5:00–6:00 P.M. | Better know as "the children's hour." Forget about yourself. Feed the baby and have a relaxing glass of wine or beer. (Great for nursing mothers!) Refresh makeup. |
| 7:00 P.M. | Eat a well-balanced dinner. Stay away from sweet desserts. They're not great for your skin, and won't do anything for your figure either. |
| 9:00 P.M. | Shower, wash hair. Use an instant conditioner. |
| 10:00 P.M. | Feed baby. Cleanse face and apply eye cream and night cream. Get into bed and go to sleep—for your health *and* your beauty. |

## WHEN YOU HAVE A MINUTE

You've probably already discovered by now that you don't have large blocks of time to spend on yourself the way you used to. However, there are odd moments when you suddenly find yourself free—while you're waiting twenty minutes for the baby to wake up from his nap, or two minutes for the nipples to be sterilized. Here are some good things to do for the skin if you have a free minute or two:

*One Minute.* Do one of the following:

- Wash your face and put on moisturizer.
- Rub body cream on rough elbows or knees.
- Rub cuticle cream on nails and cuticles.
- Apply a thick coat of clear lip-gloss.
- Spritz on a refreshing cologne.

*Five Minutes.* Do one of the following:

- Shave your legs after applying baby lotion.
- File your nails.
- Tweeze your eyebrows.

*Ten Minutes.* Do one of the following:

- Take a bath with a handful of sea salt added to the water.
- Give yourself a yogurt mask. Simply apply plain yogurt from the container to your face and leave on for 10 minutes. Rinse off with tepid water.
- If you are nursing, take off your bra or let down the flaps to expose your breasts to the air.
- Relax and put your feet up. Let your whole body relax and go limp. Let your mind go blank.
- Make a list of beauty items you need.

*Thirty Minutes.* Do one of the following:

- Play with makeup. Try to copy the latest beauty look in the magazines.
- Organize your cosmetics. Put away colors you never wear, but don't throw them away. They'll look new to you when you discover them again in a few months.
- Give yourself a manicure.

*Sixty Minutes.* If you have a babysitter do one of the following:

- Get a professional facial at a beauty salon. Have your eyelashes dyed at the same time.
- Get a massage.
- Have your legs waxed. In the summer have the bikini line done too.
- Get a professional manicure.

*A Free Morning or Afternoon.* Again if you have a babysitter, visit a salon and have all of the above done, plus:

- Take an exercise class.
- Have your hair washed and styled.

## TWO-FERS; OR, HOW TO BABY YOURSELF

When you're buying the baby's toiletries, you can often save money by supplying your own beauty product needs. Check the baby's tray for goodies such as baby powder, baby wipes, or petroleum jelly. You'll be surprised at how many baby products will double for you. Here are some uses we have discovered.

- *Petroleum Jelly.* This can be used as a night cream. A natural product, it is one of the best and safest moisture-sealers around. Petroleum jelly is also great for the dry, cracked lips nursing mothers often develop. Use it to remove makeup as well.
- *Baby Powder.* Sprinkle some glorious-smelling baby powder on after a bath or shower. It will help to absorb some of the extra perspiration that you have at this time. A warning: don't surround yourself with a big cloud of talcum. Inhaling it can be harmful to the lungs. On the baby too, use it sparingly and in an open space.
- *Baby Shampoo.* This mild shampoo is perfect if you wash your hair every day.
- *Baby Oil.* Pour a capful of this pure oil in your bath water. Baby oil is cheaper than many fancy bath oils. But it has perfume additives so wait till your postpartum checkup to try it.
- *Baby Lotion.* You can use baby lotion on your legs for shaving. Just slather it on and run the razor up your legs, wiping off excess lotion and stubble as necessary. You'll be amazed at how silky your legs feel after using this product. It's also a perfect body and hand lotion.
- *Baby Wipes.* These little towelettes which contain baby oil (never use the ones with alcohol) are great for removing eye makeup.
- *Cotton-tipped Swabs.* These are effective for catching little flecks of mascara that fall on your cheek. They're also terrific for smuding and softening eye makeup.

## POSTPARTUM PERFUME

You may have noticed that the hormone changes of pregnancy affected the way a perfume smelled on your body. Your favorite scent may continue to smell different while you nurse, so have fun experimenting with new colognes now. But remember that both nursing and bottle-feeding require a great deal of physical intimacy with the baby, whose very acute sense of smell helps the infant distinguish its mother from other adults. Researchers feel that the smelling and sniffing that goes on between the mother and the baby (and the father and the baby) is a very important part of the bonding of the human family. Use light colognes when you go out if you like, but avoid camouflaging your own smell with heavy fragrances. To your baby, your scent is the most lovely perfume in the world.

## NAIL NEWS

Remember those pretty, long, healthy nails you grew (or were supposed to have grown!) during pregnancy? Expect them to go into a bit of a slump after the baby arrives. The price for nine months of extra sturdiness must be paid. Within two to four months after the birth of your baby—as your keratin-boosting pregnancy hormones decrease—they may become brittle and break more easily. However, six months to a year after the baby, your nails will probably regain their prepregnancy strength.

You can help stop nail breakage with faithful care. Keep these suggestions in mind:

- Keep your nails shortish while they are so brittle. This is also safer for handling a new baby. File them into oval shapes to give them sturdy structures.
- Use a nail hardener or a polish with strengthening fibers.
- Choose a clear or pale shade of polish. Dark colors tend to shrink the nails.
- Use rubber gloves whenever you have to put your hands in hot water. Before putting on rubber gloves, massage a little petroleum jelly into the cuticles and nails. The heat from the gloves will activate the vaseline. Cotton gloves can be used for doing such household chores as dusting.
- Always use hand cream after putting your nails in water.

- Use a cuticle cream at night.
- Nails tend to be more brittle and to dry out in the winter when there is less humidity. Use a humidifier. It is terrific for the baby, your plants, your furniture, *and* your nails.

AT HOME OR AT THE OFFICE:

- Use a pencil or other instrument to dial the telephone. Never use your finger.
- When picking up change from the counter, instead of using your fingertips, slide the coins to the edge and push them off into the palm of your hand.
- Type with the balls of your fingers. Try to avoid hitting the keys with your nails.
- Never use your fingernails to pry open bobby pins or jewelry.
- Use your knuckle to push elevator buttons.

## PRETTY FEET

As a new mother, you are going to be on your feet a lot. Whether you are working at an office or staying at home, your baby will demand that you be on your feet and running many hours of the day—but if you can manage it, the best solution for tired feet is to periodically rest and elevate them. Remember, too, that the weight of pregnancy can cause you to gain a whole shoe size. Your prepregnancy shoes may be too tight, so have your feet measured if you're buying a new pair. If you have persistent foot problems you should have your feet checked by a podiatrist.

If your feet get very tired and sore, try the hot and cold foot baths suggested on p. 37.

If your feet get very tired easily, they may need strengthening. Try these exercises. Stand with your bare feet flat on the floor and raise up onto your toes. Stay there to the count of five and slowly lower your heels. Repeat ten times. Picking up baby rattles or other objects with your toes is another good exercise for the feet.

A friend of ours shared an old Persian recipe with us for rough skin on the feet. Pour 1 teaspoon sugar in the palm of your hand. Add enough olive oil to make a paste. Gently rub into heel, soles, and sides of feet. Rinse off. The sugar acts as an abrasive to remove dry, dead skin cells and the olive oil is a great lubricator. This leaves the skin on your feet feeling smooth.

As a lovely luxury, get a professional pedicure, or give yourself one. Once you have the prettiest feet in town, invest in a pair of romantic evening sandals. Consider a pair in gold or silver. Next: book a babysitter and tell your husband you're both going dancing!

## THE FIVE-MINUTE MAKEUP ROUTINE

The theme for makeup and beauty care after you have your baby is speed. Here, Liz O'Brien, a model, shows us her new, streamlined daytime makeup routine. "It takes all of five minutes and succeeds in making me feel better all day long," says Liz. "If I let myself hang around wearing a bathrobe and no makeup, I feel like a frump. These five minutes out of my day boost my spirits one hundred percent!"

Liz knows that for your skin to look its brightest and healthiest during your first nine months postpartum, you will have to pamper it the way you pamper your baby—with lots of love and care and . . . yes, time. Unfortunately there are no magic lotions to put on the skin that can make up for what you lack inside. New motherhood brings with it a lot of fatigue, stress, and poor diet habits. All these can cause pale, drawn skin, dark circles under the eyes, oily skin, and even acne.

Good health habits are the foundation of good looks. Skin is the litmus paper for your habits, showing the effects of stress and deficiencies in rest and good diet almost immediately. Some problems are inevitable and you can temporarily camouflage with facials, masks, and makeup. But try to restore good health habits to your life as soon as possible.

Once your life becomes balanced again, your skin will probably glow like your baby's. Add makeup daily, and you'll be as pretty as ever, or even prettier.

# · A NEWBORN BEAUTY ROUTINE ·

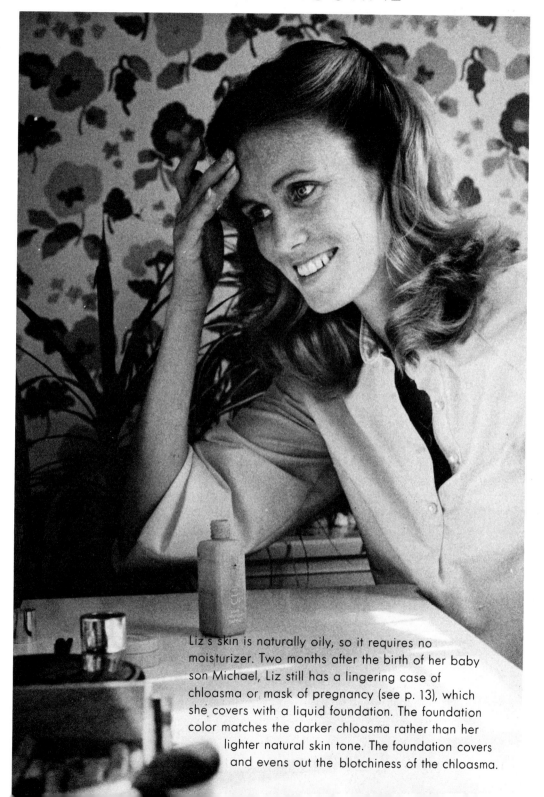

Liz's skin is naturally oily, so it requires no moisturizer. Two months after the birth of her baby son Michael, Liz still has a lingering case of chloasma or mask of pregnancy (see p. 13), which she covers with a liquid foundation. The foundation color matches the darker chloasma rather than her lighter natural skin tone. The foundation covers and evens out the blotchiness of the chloasma.

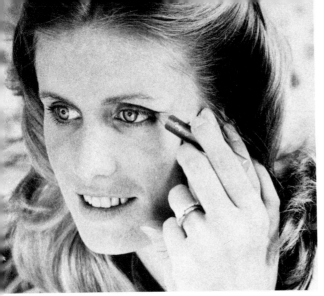

Next Liz uses one of her three favorite eyeshadow crayons. Her daytime shades are taupe, pewter gray, and mauve. Here she uses the taupe to cover the entire lid. Then, under her lower lashes she draws a soft line of color from the outer corner to the center. Liz also wears mascara during the day. With a dark brown shade she coats the top side of her upper lashes first and then the underside. She repeats the process for her lower lashes.

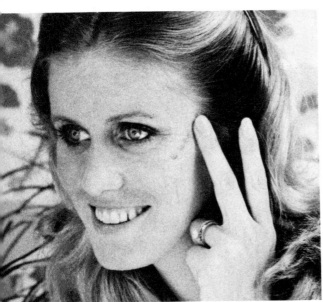

Liz likes the soft look of a liquid rouge for daytime. She places three small dots on her cheekbones inclining upward toward the temples. She carefully blends the rouge into the foundation. If Liz has been up with the baby all night, the color helps camouflage the drawn look of fatigue.

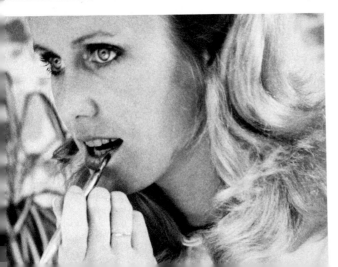

A mulberry lip gloss is applied with a brush for the final touch.

*Opposite page:* A pretty new mother! Although the day ahead might be a busy one, Liz is ready. She will surprise any unannounced visitors, looking pretty and natural even with the demands of being a full-time mother.

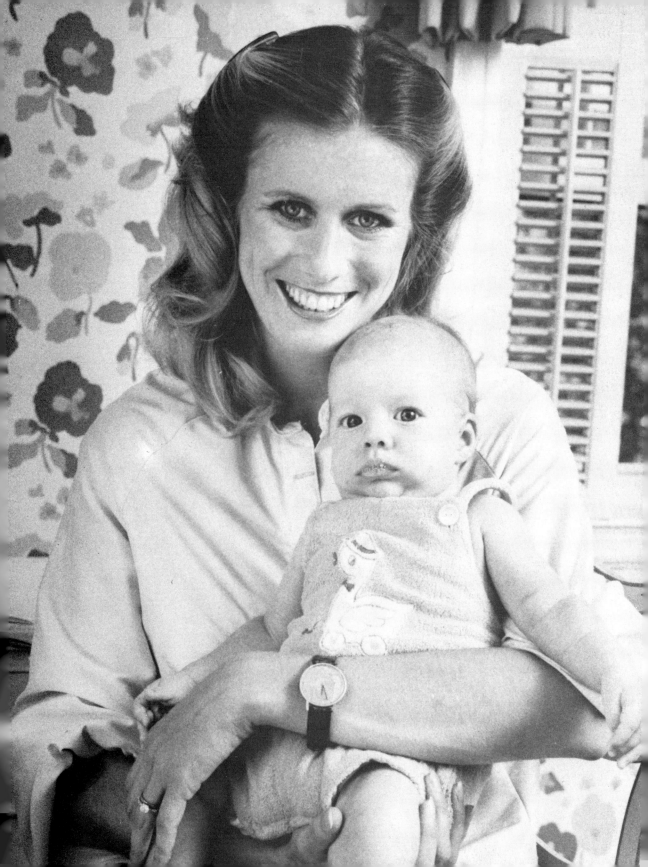

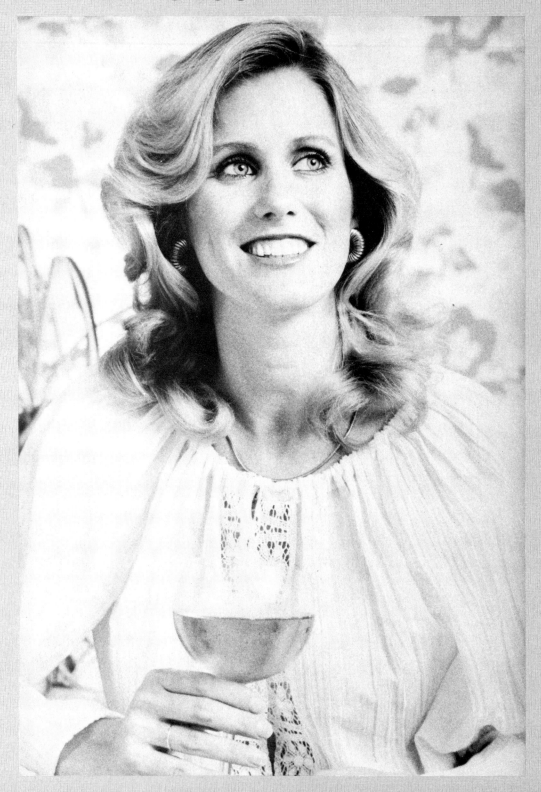

For those essential evenings out Liz gives herself a little more time for makeup. She has the babysitter come a half-hour early to allow ample time to give herself a dazzling evening look. If Liz looks and feels very tired, she uses the following exercises to restore color to her face. She gets on to her hands and knees on her bed. She then lowers her head to the bed and holds that position for one minute. This exercise also stretches and relaxes the muscles in the neck and back. Liz then starts out with her five-minute daytime makeup routine, minus her daytime lip gloss. She adds from there:

**under eyes** A second coat of foundation to cover circles. (At the end of a long day Liz's fatigue often shows here.)

**eyes** Liz lines her eyes with a dark brown liquid eyeliner, which she softly smudges with a cotton-tipped swab. She uses a gray pencil to line the inner edge of the lower lid. For evening Liz extends her mauve eyeshadow right up to the brow, lightening as she approaches the brow. She uses a light brown pencil to fill in her eyebrows.

**cheeks** On top of her liquid rouge, Liz uses a rose powder blusher.

**lips** First, Liz outlines her lips in red pencil. She then brightens her whole look with a cherry-red lipstick, blending it into the pencil outline. Over this she uses a clear lip gloss.

**final touch** Liz dips a big brush into a box of very fine talcum powder, shakes the excess, and lightly dusts her face. This extra touch gives a beautiful, even-finished, matte look. Here she is, lovely and ready to go.

# CHAPTER·XII·
# Hair—Quick Solutions to New-Mother Problems

"EVERY TIME I BRUSH MY HAIR, I wind up with an amazing amount of hair in my brush. What is happening?"

"Will all the hair I'm now losing grow back?"

"My hair is straighter since I've had my baby. Is this permanent?"

"Is there any reason that I should avoid certain hair care products while I'm breastfeeding?"

Although your hair may have looked its best and healthiest during your pregnancy, after the baby's birth it is a whole new story.

Hair loss or newly straight hair are two problems you may have to cope with for the first time; in addition, you'll discover you don't have the time you used to have for washing and styling. But take heart—our talks with hair-care specialists, stylists, and women like you have yielded marvelous advice on how to find time for and streamline your hair care, what to do for postpartum hair problems, and how to babyproof your hair.

## WHY IS MY HAIR FALLING OUT?

Abby had heard of hair loss after having a baby but never expected to see her hair actually matting the drain after each shampoo. "I stopped washing

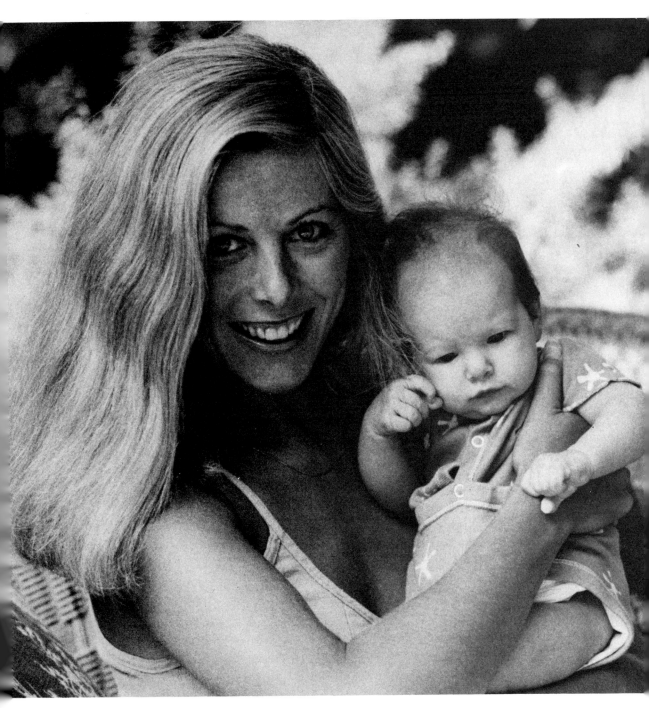

Six-week-old Sophie can't resist the touch of Joanne's freshly washed hair.

and brushing my hair for a week at a time. I'd only comb it a little to put it in place." With all her precautions, Abby's hair continued to thin for about six weeks. "By then," said Abby, "I felt like I had half of what I used to have. My husband said he couldn't see the difference. But I think he was just being nice." Within eight months, however, Abby saw new hair grow back, as do most women who experience hair loss.

Almost all women will lose some hair in the three to six months after they have their babies. This syndrome, called postpartum alopecia, is actually a reaction to the full and lovely head of hair you had while you were pregnant. During pregnancy (see pp. 47–51) your hair continues to grow while the normal falling-out stage is arrested. But upon delivery, your hair is suddenly thrown into the "catagen" or "transitional" phase during which the hair shrinks and ceases its production of keratin. This lasts for a few weeks. Then the "telogen" or "resting" phase occurs, during which the follicles stop shrinking and rest. They rest for about three months before they are finally dislodged by brushing or washing—which is why hair loss occurs three or so months after delivery, rather than immediately.

What all this means is that you're losing more hairs *after* pregnancy because you lost fewer *during* pregnancy. While normal hair loss is between 70 and 150 hairs a day, during postpartum alopecia you will lose between 500 and 600 a day. But, as Dr. Jonathan Zizmor in his book *Superhair* (see Bibliography) remarks, "Actually (hair loss due to childbirth) is a positive sign, since the falling hair is usually being pushed out by . . . new growth."

Hairdressers and dermatologists report that women who don't know about this postpartum phenomenon come to their offices and salons frightened, depressed, and sometimes crying. Since hair has historically been the symbol of strength, beauty, and sexual attractiveness, losing hair is a traumatic experience. (Balding among men often has a devastating psychological effect.)

Some women, on the other hand, notice no difference in their hair from pregnancy to postpartum. This doesn't mean they're not losing hair. Dermatologist Dr. Norman Orentreich tells us that we can, at any time, take thinning scissors, thin our hair twenty to thirty percent all over, and never notice a difference. Whether you think you've lost a lot or a little, remember that for most people it will all grow back. Of course, hair does tend to thin as we get older anyway, and for a few of us, pregnancy accelerates this process. But *permanent* hair loss from postpartum alopecia is very rare.

If you still feel you're losing too much hair, see a dermatologist. You may have another condition that pregnancy sometimes triggers, androgenic alopecia. This condition is inherited, so check with your female relatives. If you aren't nursing, your doctor can treat you with hormones to slow down hair loss.

## "WHAT CAN I DO FOR 'SKINNY HAIR'?"

Postpartum alopecia may have thinned out your hair a little or a lot. Even though your thinner hair is just temporary, you should know some facts about caring for it during this special time. For perhaps the first time in your life, you may have to be creative about plumping your hair. Take this test to see how much you know about hair care for hair loss, and use the information in the answers to help care for your skinnier head of hair.

Mark "true" or "false" after each statement.

|  | T | F |
|---|---|---|
| 1. Frequent shampooing causes you to lose more hair than if you wash only once a week. | ☐ | ☐ |
| 2. Protein conditioners can change hair noticeably. | ☐ | ☐ |
| 3. Blow dryers, electric rollers, and curling irons accelerate hair loss. | ☐ | ☐ |
| 4. Vigorous brushing stimulates the hair and encourages hair growth. | ☐ | ☐ |
| 5. Hair coloring makes hair look thicker. | ☐ | ☐ |
| 6. A layered hair cut makes thin hair look fuller. | ☐ | ☐ |
| 7. Wearing hair in a ponytail or topknot increases hair loss. | ☐ | ☐ |
| 8. Special vitamins will make hair grow. | ☐ | ☐ |

ANSWERS

1. *True.* The stress of shampooing does cause hair to fall out more rapidly. However, you would lose the same amount of hair eventually. Do use a mild shampoo while you are losing hair. Lather only once and rinse thoroughly. Shampooing is actually very good for the hair because it stimulates the scalp, removes excess sebum, and helps the hair follicles function so that new hair will be healthy. Clean hair appears fuller. It is not flattened down with dirt and grease and it has more air in it. Highlights and shine from shampooing contribute to the overall appearance of health. So don't avoid shampooing and brushing your hair. You will lose hair *sooner* but you won't lose *more*—and your whole look will improve.

2. *True.* Conditioners containing body-building ingredients such as protein and balsam can coat the strands of hair, strengthening them and making them thicker. Protein also makes hair shine by smoothing down the cuticle of each hair. Conditioning your hair prevents breakage by eliminating snarls and tangles. Remember to use a wide-toothed comb on wet hair. Allow it to dry a little first and then comb to minimize hair loss.

3. *False.* Unless your hair is very dry and brittle. In this case avoid electric rollers, curling irons, and blow dryers. If your hair is normal, and you use these electric wonders properly, they will not cause your hair to fall out. To insure this:

   - Don't use electric rollers every day.
   - Always use end papers with electric rollers.
   - Don't use electric rollers on wet hair.
   - Remove electric rollers gently. Don't pull.
   - If you use a curling iron, make sure it is coated with teflon.
   - Before blow-drying thin hair, comb hair through with wide-toothed comb as mentioned above, then move dryer freely all over hair till hair is almost dry.
   - Use a natural bristle brush and dryer to smooth down the top layer only. This gives thin hair more volume.

4. *False.* Vigorous combing and brushing can put a great strain on hair and

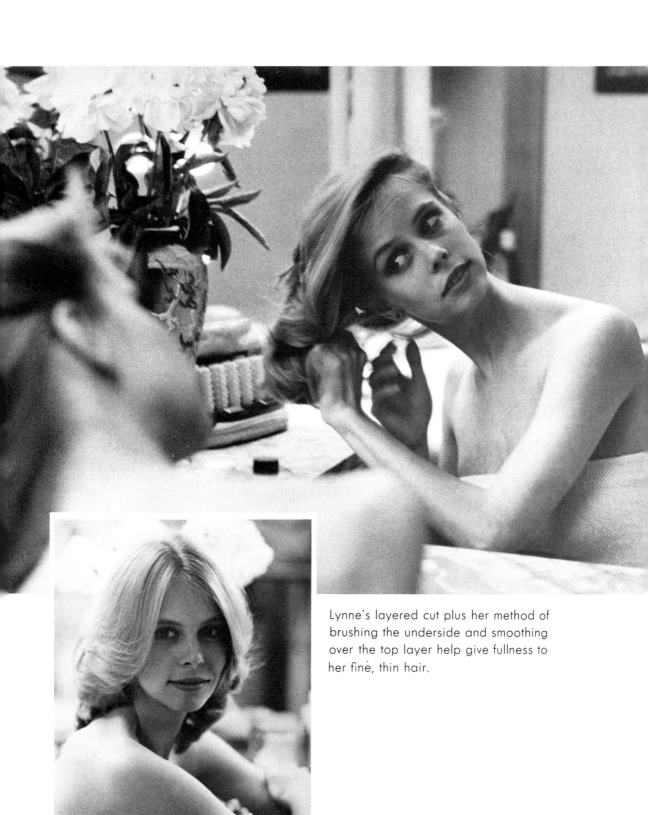

Lynne's layered cut plus her method of
brushing the underside and smoothing
over the top layer help give fullness to
her fine, thin hair.

can actually pull out and break hair. To remove tangles and style, use a natural bristle brush through hair only once. To make hair look fuller, throw hair forward and brush down. Flip head back and smooth just the top layer, as Lynne does on p. 299.

5. *True.* Coloring hair will actually increase the diameter of each hair strand, and your whole head of hair will look thicker. Coloring is therefore a good solution for thin hair. If you don't want to change your color, choose a shade close to your own. Warning: if your hair has the tendency to break easily, coloring could make it worse.

6. *True.* A layered cut will add fullness. This cut is usually wash and wear, too, making it an ideal postpartum style. Layered cuts are not good, however, for stick-straight fine hair. This type of hair needs volume and a blunt cut works best.

7. *True.* The constant pulling of the hair can cause it to fall out. Always make sure the ponytail or topknot does not pull the roots of your hair. Use covered rubber bands for these styles to prevent further breakage.

8. *False.* There are no vitamins to make your hair grow. You do need a balanced diet to get all the vitamins and minerals needed for a good head of hair. A lack of these essential vitamins and minerals in your diet will slow hair growth, and make hair brittle and lackluster. Don't waste your money on vitamins.

## BIRTH CONTROL PILLS AND HAIR GROWTH

Margie wanted to start birth control pills for the first time eight months after she had her son Phillip. However, she heard they cause problems with hair growth and loss and, since she'd lost a lot of hair after she had her baby, she was hesitant.

Actually, birth control pills mimic pregnancy in that they add hormones, especially estrogen, to your system. Your hair (and skin) often benefit from this hormone, the way they do during pregnancy. Then, when you stop the pill, you may experience hair loss just as you do after you have your baby. If your doctor approves, and you are not nursing, it's fine to resume birth control pills. The effect on your hair will be beneficial.

## TEXTURAL CHANGES IN YOUR HAIR

Aside from the hair loss phenomenon, most women see no change in their hair. However, in our interviews about twenty percent reported some change in condition or texture.

"I had frizzy hair all my life before I had Danielle," said a twenty-one-year-old mother of an eleven-month-old girl. "My hair now has long, lanky curls. It's still wavy, but it's straightened considerably."

Pierre Ouaknine of the Pierre Michel Coiffures in New York, observed, "I've seen hair go from curly to straight, with the exception being black women. I've never seen their hair change after having a baby. And I've never seen straight hair turn curly after pregnancy." (In our interviews we did uncover one case of straight hair turning wavy.) Usually these changes in hair texture are permanent. With age, curly hair tends to straighten, and pregnancy seems to advance this metamorphosis.

However, for some women the change is only temporary. "I had long, naturally curly hair when I had my first baby a couple of years ago," said Dorothy, mother of a two-year-old. "Within two months after giving birth, my hair went stick-straight! I don't know if it was fatigue, since I'd been up night after night with the baby, or simply the hormonal changes. After about six months my curls returned and my hair looked the same as it did before I got pregnant."

If the texture of your hair is different after delivery, discuss the change with your hairdresser. Your new look may be welcome.

## SHORTCUTS TO BEAUTIFUL HAIR

"I wish there were some little gnome who could come along each day and prick me to let me know it's time to wash my hair," said Louise, complaining about priorities when her baby was six weeks old. "You *have* to feed the baby but you *can* let your hair go one more day without washing it. But tired, dirty hair makes me feel and look awful!"

Louise's plight is almost universal. Hairdresser Didier Malige said of brand-new mothers in his salon: "They seem to be so concerned about time. It's all they can talk about." As a bachelor he didn't understand that babies, and consequently mothers, are on tight schedules. Even if you have help with the new baby and the rest of the family, washing your hair, putting on makeup, and dressing so you don't look like a hausfrau take a *lot* of energy. But a clean, shiny, pretty head of hair is probably what will make you feel the best.

Hair care is one of the beauty aspects you can control. You may still have some of that extra weight you gained and not be able to wear your prepregnancy jeans, but if your hair looks good, *you* look good. And you can make it happen:

- If mornings are too busy, try washing your hair at night when the baby is asleep. Even though you are tired at night, the extra ten minutes spent washing your hair will be worth it. Towel dry your hair or let it dry naturally if blow-drying seems too exhausting. Write thank-you notes, watch TV, or talk to your husband while it dries.
- If you are used to applying shampoo to your hair two or three times, try sudsing just once or twice. Often the thought of two or three applications and two or three rinse-offs is overwhelming. Use an instant conditioner or cream rinse to relax hair. This cuts time combing and untangling your hair.
- If the water pressure in your shower is poor, rinsing can take a tortuously long time. Invest in a new nozzle or showerhead so the pressure of the water, not your hands, does most of the rinsing work. You will be amazed at how your attitude towards shampooing changes once this time-saving nozzle is installed.
- Set up and stick to a schedule of shampooing and, if you need it, styling with a blow dryer or curlers. This can be done every day, every other day, or every three days, in accordance with your needs.
- Use electric rollers for a fast (five- to ten-minute) hair set. If you've

never used them before, now is the time to invest in a set. Sleeping overnight on rollers is dreadful, whether you are a new mother or not. To help preserve some of the curl when you go to bed, pin hair up in large curls with bobby pins, or try catching up long blunt-cut hair in a ponytail on top of your head and setting with two or three large rollers. A ponytail also works without the rollers—just roll it under several times and fasten it with big bobby pins. The trick is to get the hair on the top of your head instead of flattening it on the sides of your head while you sleep. If you have curly or wavy hair, try putting it in braids before you sleep. Unbraid and comb out into waves in the morning.

- Don't think that you must set your hair each time you wash it. As long as it is clean, hair looks fine pulled back with a ribbon or caught up with a comb.
- Many beauty salons offer discount wash and sets, usually in the middle of the week, without an appointment. Watch for these specials. Hire a babysitter and slip away one afternoon or after work and have someone else shampoo and set your hair.

## BABYPROOF HAIRSTYLES

Try pulling your long hair out of an infant's clenched fist, and you learn a new respect for the strength of your little toughie. Your loose swinging hair is fair game for babies, so you take your risks in wearing it down. Why not try one of these styles for pretty ways to get your hair up and out of the way of grabby little hands?

In the chaos of your rapidly changing life, a natural instinct is to want to hold onto some part of your prepregnancy self. And your old hairstyle seems to be one of the things women are most tenacious about. But don't let this very natural fear of change hold you back from trying new and flattering hairstyles. Whether it's been the highlighting you've wanted to do, getting your long hair layered, having a professional protein treatment, or adorning your hair with a fresh flower, change can make you even more exciting and provocative in your new role.

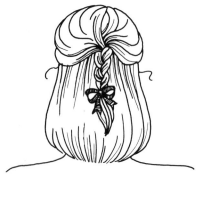

A variation on a classic style pulls back the crown and sides of your hair into a braid secured with a covered rubber band.

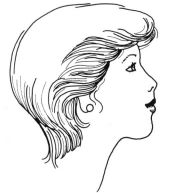

If you were thinking about trying a short cut before you had your baby but held off because you were afraid it would make the pregnant you look like a pinhead, do it now! A short style will keep your hair out of the reach of tiny fingers. The one shown here gives a little volume and is easy to care for with simple shampooing and blow-drying.

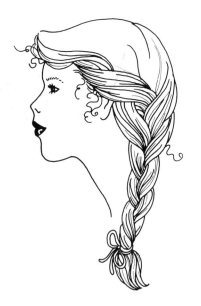

Hair is also easily kept out of baby's reach by putting it into one long braid or a pretty ponytail placed high on your head.

# • ALVA'S FRENCH SNAIL •

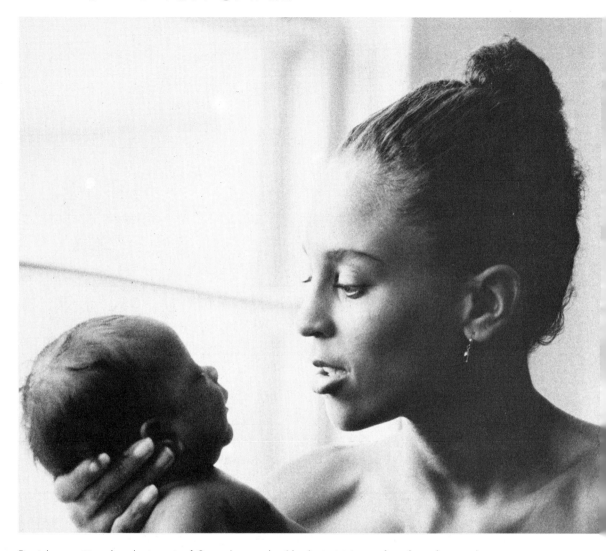

Besides getting her hair out of Soma's reach, Alva's twist is perfect for after a shower, sunbathing, or exercising, to get hair off the neck and into a cool style. Alva simply puts her hair into the classic "French twist" by pulling it back, twisting it to one side, and securing it with hairpins. However, in Alva's version, she pulls the twist upward, so the effect is more like a snail. The hair left over on top is then tucked under with straight pins. (Alva prefers plastic to metal hairpins because she feels they are less likely to damage her dry hair.) Alva's style is easy and pretty for any new mother.

# · JOANNE'S WET LOOK ·

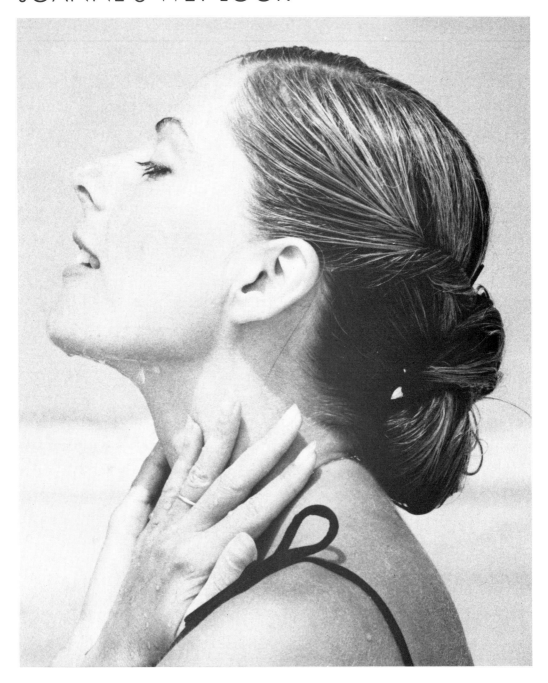

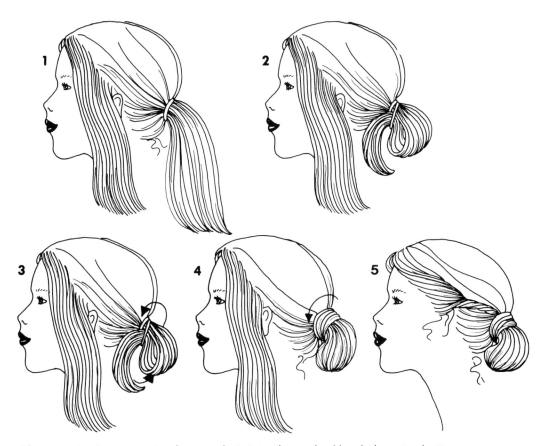

After a swim Joanne twists her wet hair into this style. Here's how to do it:

1. Part your hair on the side and section off pieces of hair on both sides of your head. Let this hair hang loose while you do the rest of the styling. Then pull the rest of your hair into a ponytail about two inches from the nape of your neck and secure with a covered rubber band.

2. Loop your ponytail up and pull the end through the covered rubber band one more time so that half of the ponytail is caught up by the elastic and the end hangs down loose.

3. Pull the section of hair left out of the ponytail up and twist it over and around the covered rubber band.

4. Secure it underneath with hairpins or bobby pins.

5. Next, twist the side pieces neatly and pull them back to meet the top of the ponytail. Tuck the ends under the loop and secure them with hairpins so that the ends cannot be seen.

# CHAPTER ·XIII·
# Sex—After You've Had Your Baby

WRITE DOWN "TRUE" OR "FALSE" after the following statements:

1. "After my episiotomy heals and the soreness has disappeared, there's no reason I can't start enjoying sex."
2. "Sexual intercourse for the first time after the baby is born always hurts. There's no way except a little praying to prepare for the first time."
3. "Childbirth permanently damages the vaginal muscles. Sex will never be as good as it once was."
4. "Nursing mothers feel sexier sooner than nonnursing mothers."
5. "A new mother's sex drive always returns to what it was before she got pregnant about six weeks after the baby is born."
6. "Husbands don't mind the ban on sex for a while after birth."
7. "There's not much to be done to put romance back in your life for the first few months, since the baby is taking up so much time and effort."

## IS THERE SEX AFTER BABY?

If you answered "false" to all of these questions—or found yourself saying, "It ain't necessarily so!" to each of them, you've either already had a baby or

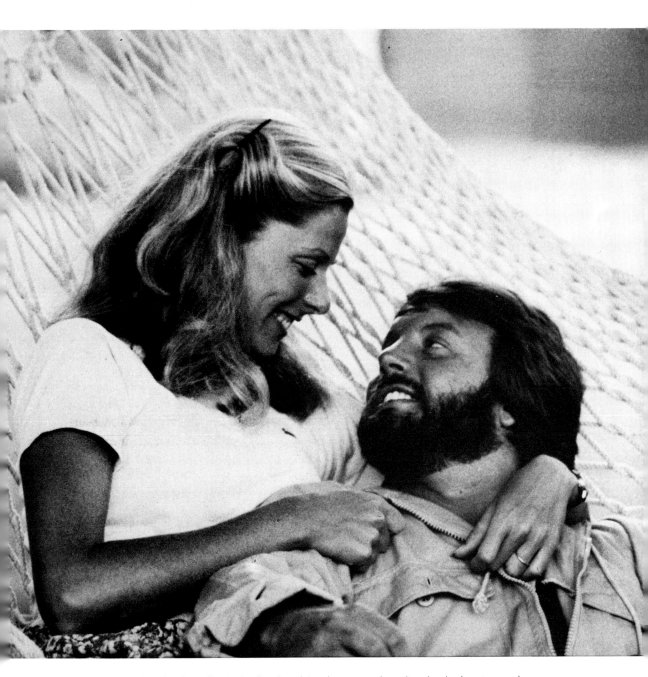

Joanne and her husband, Mick, this book's photographer, let the babysitter take over the two children so that they can have some time to spend alone together.

know a lot more about postpartum sex than the rest of us. Sex life after the baby is born is a much-neglected subject—but it is tremendously important. The women we interviewed shared information on when sex can be resumed, what it's like the first time afterward, sex and the nursing mother, why you may feel a diminished sex drive at first, how to avoid feeling negative about yourself, how not to neglect your husband at this time, and, finally, how to put romance back in your life. This can be a difficult period in your and your husband's life—but time, knowledge, and each couple's willingness to communicate will do wonders. Read on.

## "WHEN CAN I RESUME SEX?"

*Joe:* "How soon can you start having sex again after the baby's born?"
*Frank:* "Depends on whether you've got a private or semiprivate room."

Only a man could have come up with this joke—any woman would wince at the thought. Naturally, after giving birth, your vagina and the muscles of the perineum have been stretched. The vagina and labia swell so much from this trauma and from your episiotomy that they can often be felt as you walk during the first two or three days after birth. This should go away within a few days, but obviously, immediate intercourse is out.

How soon after the birth of your baby *can* you resume sex? The answer is: when your obstetrician gives the okay. More liberal doctors ask you to wait about four weeks, while the conservative ones ask you to wait until your six-week postpartum checkup.

After the second or third week, you can have sex outside of the vagina. Since you'll still be secreting lochia, oral sex is probably undesirable. But masturbation, manual stimulation, and orgasms are fine as long as nothing enters the vagina.

If you don't want to wait six weeks for intercourse, ask for a four-week postpartum checkup. Most doctors are happy to comply. Many doctors don't give you a specific time limit and some women start sex sooner than their postpartum checkup. This is not advisable. If your doctor hasn't said when you can resume sexual intercourse, ask her, preferably in the presence of your husband. Medical conditions are different for each woman. Women who have delivered by Caesarean section are usually asked to wait six weeks.

Why are you asked to abstain from sex for as long as six weeks after childbirth? Doctors we interviewed list the following reasons:

1. The episiotomy must heal correctly. Although the first layers of skin usually heal in five to six days, the underlying tissues do not heal for three to four weeks. Only your doctor's examination can determine your progress. Meanwhile, it is important not to tear this mending by having sexual intercourse. The soreness in the area must also disappear.
2. The vaginal canal has undergone changes which affect its bacterial makeup. Its microorganisms must redevelop to protect the vagina and internal system from foreign bacteria introduced by the penis and/or the seminal fluid.
3. The cervix must be completely closed and the cervical mucus glands must be functioning in order to prevent uterine infection. This is also true for Caesarean section women.

The long ban on sexual intercourse can give rise to a host of problems, especially when love and affection are expressed only with sexual intercourse. If you are asked to refrain from sexual intercourse six weeks before and six weeks after the birth of your baby, this means three months of denying yourself and your loved one, one of life's greatest pleasures—and all the other implications of an active sex life, such as reassurance of physical attractiveness and ongoing proof of a man's virility or a woman's femininity. So where does this leave you when you're dying to hug, hold, and have tender sex with your husband? Well, you *can* hug and you can caress and *be* caressed everywhere except in the perineal area. (Women who have had a Caesarean section, however, must be careful not to touch or put pressure on their stitches.) The need to be held and reassured is stronger than ever in the initial postpartum period. If—as during pregnancy—you and your husband can expand your sexual expression to include warm looks, kisses, and hugs, both of you will feel more comfortable and emotionally reassured during this trying period.

After six weeks, many women still don't feel sufficiently energetic, comfortable, or sexually aroused to resume sex. Once your obstetrician has given the okay, try to show your husband that you still care for him. Even if your sex life is not the same for six months, expressing your love sexually is sometimes the easiest way to communicate to your partner that you love him. If you're right back on course, and loving sex within three to six weeks, great. If not, don't worry—you're not alone. Most sexual problems, such as slow arousal, inability to reach orgasm, etc., correct themselves within these first six months.

## THE FIRST TIME

"Making love the first time with Dorothy after we'd had our baby was one of the strangest and most spiritual experiences of my life," said John. "Having physical proof of our lovemaking ten months ago in the room next door gave me a whole new feeling about sex, its magnitude and its implications."

For men, this first time may be spiritual. But for women, the first usually causes some pain. "I wish my doctor had warned me!" said Rosina, a Latin American beauty, after her first baby. "I was so frightened by the pain I called my doctor right away. 'Oh that passes after a few times,' he cheerfully told me, 'just keep practicing.'" Many doctors don't prepare their patients well for first-time intercourse after the baby is born. Many problems could be avoided if couples did a little preliminary work.

As soon as three to four weeks after the delivery, you and/or your husband can start preparing for intercourse. Using a lubricant jelly or cream, insert one finger into your vagina and move it around, gently pressing against the walls of the vagina. Repeat the procedure with two fingers and then three fingers. Do this exercise many times to dilate the vagina before you have intercourse for the first time.

Talk to your husband before you resume sexual relations. Make sure he understands the delicate condition of your perineal area and your fears, if you have any, about resuming sex. Don't feel you have to rush right into vaginal sex. There are plenty of alternatives (see p. 183). When your doctor has given the go-ahead for resuming intercourse, remember these points:

- Go *slowly* at first. Have your husband repeat the vaginal stretching exercises above. He should be able to insert three fingers before attempting intercourse. Don't worry about the time delay. Enjoy the closeness. You can always bring each other to orgasm with manual or oral stimulation.

- If you still feel a little sore when your husband touches you, your doctor can prescribe a topical anesthetic, perhaps the one you used on your episiotomy stitches and/or hemorrhoids in the hospital, to apply before intercourse.

- Spend a lot of time fondling, caressing, and touching. Many women are naturally nervous about possible pain. This causes you to contract your vagina and makes it even more difficult when attempting intercourse. Gentle foreplay will help you relax. Kegel exercises may also give you control here, allowing you to relax your vagina. In *Human Sexual Response,* sex researchers Masters and Johnson report that—in a study of six women—the subjects did not respond as quickly or intensely as usual to sexual stimulation in the period after birth. Don't be discouraged if the fireworks are slow to take off.

- Use the female-superior position so that you can control the penetration of the penis. The face-to-face position on your sides is also recommended since penetration is not very deep. This position is also recommended for Caesarean section women since the scar is subjected to less pressure. Rear entry and anal intercourse are not recommended for the first times since these positions create too much pressure on the episiotomy.

- Use a lubricant for the first penetration by the penis. Ask your husband to be very gentle and careful. Keep trying—it gets better every time.

## BIRTH CONTROL

For even the first time, you should use birth control! It is possible that you could become pregnant, even while nursing. Despite the traditional wisdom that nursing suppresses ovulation, the facts are otherwise. Even if you don't have your period, you may be ovulating.

Your obstetrician will suggest the best birth control method for you. A lubricated condom to be used along with contraceptive foam is often recommended. Doctors may recommend birth control pills for nonnursing mothers but usually hesitate when a mother is lactating. A doctor usually likes to wait three months postpartum for complete involution before fitting you for a new diaphragm, as your size may have changed with the birth of your baby. Intrauterine devices, however, are often inserted during the first postpartum visit.

If you have elected not to have any more children, you might consider a tubal ligation to permanently arrest your reproduction capacity. Many women have this simple procedure done while still in the hospital after the birth. However, many authorities now suggest waiting eighteen months. More men are now accepting responsibility for birth control by having a vasectomy. Discuss all options with your husband and doctor.

## DOES CHILDBIRTH MAKE SEXUAL INTERCOURSE LESS ENJOYABLE?

The Caesarean-section rate in Rio de Janeiro, Brazil, is exceptionally high, especially among well-born and high income women. This, reports one American doctor, results from the belief that natural delivery babies stretch the vagina, making sex less exciting for the husband and/or the wife. Having an unnecessary Caesarean section seems frivolous enough, but is there any truth to this belief?

There is no doubt that natural deliveries do stretch vaginal and pelvic floor muscles, but changes may be temporary. Regaining full strength of these muscles is a matter of genetics and exercise. If you were born with elastic muscles, you will probably regain your original vaginal and pelvic floor strength. With exercise, even a mother of six can regain most of her original strength. In rare cases, when vaginal muscles are weak, and medical problems occur, vaginal plastic surgery can be done to tighten the vagina.

"When a wife or husband complains about 'not feeling enough' after the baby is born," said one obstetrician we interviewed, "it's usually because the couple places too much emphasis on the act of sexual intercourse itself. My wife has had four children and she is not as tight as when I first married her. However, the emotional aspects of love and feeling for the other person should be enough to make up the difference." Instead of vaginal plastic surgery for these cases, several visits to a sex or marriage counselor are recommended.

Full recovery of vaginal strength should come about within six months. Continue the Kegels! You can end up even tighter and stronger than before you had your baby!

## SEX AND THE NURSING MOTHER

How will breast-feeding affect your sex life? Each woman's body and psyche respond differently to the process of lactation. Jill told us: "I felt like the quintessential mother. I felt earthy and sexy and I felt like making love all the time. Something about nursing stirred me. In fact, I had so much love for my baby and my husband I couldn't give it often enough."

Linda's experience was just the opposite: "Nursing was absolutely exhausting for me—especially in the beginning. I was too tired for sex. Every time Barry and I made love, I'd actually be thinking that I was wasting valuable time I could be using to sleep."

One study conducted by Masters and Johnson found that, like Jill, mothers who nurse are more eager to resume sexual relations after birth than mothers who don't. In our random sampling, however, more women shared Linda's feelings.

Dr. Don Sloan, an obstetrician who has helped many couples with sexual problems, reports that there is no way to generalize about sexual feelings during the breast-feeding months. "If you study one hundred lactating women," he says, "one third will want sex less, one third will want sex more, and one third will have the same sex drive." (Approximately the same ratio of interest in sex will be true for nonnursing mothers.)

Your husband's reaction to your nursing breasts may play a part in your sexual feelings. "I felt like a pin-up for six months," said one pretty twenty-four-year-old mother, whose husband loved the look of her newly big breasts. Other men say that milk-laden breasts feel different. Some men are fascinated while other men are turned off to see their wives' breasts spurt milk after orgasm. Nursing might desensitize the nipple and breast area, but this is usually temporary. If it inhibits your response, move attention away from the breast area during lovemaking.

Besides leaking milk and desensitized nipples, there are other inhibitors to sex in nursing. A few nursing mothers will find their vaginas lubricate less during sexual intercourse. Dr. Sloan reports that for nursing women "our studies have verified a little later resumption of the physiologic lubrication—a true six-week delay." Indeed, a number of breast-feeding women do not feel their prepregnancy "normal" selves during sex until they've weaned. One woman said, "Within a week after weaning Daniel, I began having faster and stronger orgasms. I was finally back to my old self. It was nice!"

The simple reason why you are slow to lubricate during sex while you are nursing is that lactation tends to suppress the estrogen output in the body. Menstruation, also, is often delayed. When your period *does* return while you're nursing, your ability to lubricate during sex improves. If you're having trouble lubricating and feel sore during or after sexual intercourse, try using a lubricating jelly. This often clears up your problem immediately. Also spend more time than usual on foreplay to allow the lubrication process to begin.

Occasionally, a breast-feeding mother will not be able to lubricate at all. This was Marcia's experience. Each of the four times she and Jimmy attempted intercourse, it hurt. She knew it was supposed to be uncomfortable the first few times after the baby was born. She also knew that two of her breast-feeding friends had had similar trouble. "It's fine if the earth doesn't move," she thought, "but why does it actually hurt when he goes inside?"

Dr. Gideon Panter, in *Now That You've Had Your Baby* (see Bibliography) writes that sometimes during breast-feeding the pituitary gland does not release FSH, the ovary-stimulating hormone. "The ovary, when not stimulated, produces little or no estrogen. The vagina is one of the organs affected by estrogen, and without it the vagina frequently tightens and dries abnormally."

Dr. Panter's advice is to use a topical estrogen cream inserted with the fingers or an applicator. Some doctors prescribe low-dosage estrogen birth-control pills for this problem. These often relieve the problem but possibly have other side effects.

The strongest antiaphrodisiac you have to cope with while nursing may be exhaustion. Besides the fact that you are burning up to 1000 calories a day producing milk, you are up sometimes as often as every three hours in the middle of the night, when you first get home from the hospital and even longer if the baby has problems sleeping or digesting. Things will get better once the baby sleeps through the night, so have patience and try to catch naps during the day.

Don't force yourself to have sex but do think of your husband's needs. Many nursing mothers become so involved with their babies that their husbands feel, and actually are, excluded. The "nursing couple" of mommy and infant can be threatening to a father. "I had a much better time with the first two kids," said Bill. "Ginny is nursing our third for the first time and I feel helpless. I used to do the evening and middle-of-the-night bottle feedings. Now it's just Ginny and the baby. I'm not so sure I like this breast-feeding."

Nursing a little dependent newborn does create a very tight bond between mother and child, often with the by-product of sexual arousal. Many mothers report clitoral sensations, lubricating, and even orgasm while they're nursing. Some repress this or even wean because of it. Others enjoy it. It is thought that this sexual arousal is nature's way of making breast-feeding a pleasant experience to insure survival of the species. Be aware that this may be temporarily taking the place of sex between you and your husband. Try to get your mind off the baby for a while when you're with your husband.

## "WHY DO I FEEL SO TURNED OFF BY SEX?"

If your sex life is back to normal soon after the birth, life with the baby becomes easier sooner. But having a poor sex life, or no sex life at all, seems to magnify the problems and disruptions a new baby brings about. Why is a diminished sex drive so common during the postpartum period?

Besides fatigue, physical discomfort, and new priorities, another problem for new mothers is the conflict of images. How you look now and how you imagined you'd look might be poles apart. You may have imagined that you were going to be a cool, chic, attractive, fulfilled woman tending to your child, making other men's hearts beat as they recognized your womanliness. We are influenced by fashion magazines which glow at Christmastime with beautiful, elegant mothers in designer clothes baking gingerbread men with their equally beautiful tow-headed children in velvet suits and Mary Janes.

Instead you find yourself in the New Mother Trap. You're always wearing your old clothes because you don't want the baby to mess on your good things. You're too tired and frustrated when your husband comes home to hold a decent conversation. You have no time to spend on yourself doing all the things that used to make you feel attractive, such as polishing your nails, or doing your hair. All these are minuses in your sex life.

Do you recognize some of these complaints?

- I'm ten pounds overweight and yesterday someone asked me when I was going to have the baby.

- My bottom is so sore I've considered redecorating our house in inflatable furniture.
- I've gone partially deaf in my left ear thanks to my beautiful daughter.
- Eight straight hours of sleep is a thing of the past.
- My voluptuous breasts feel so sore and tender that I'd trade them in for a training bra in a second.
- I'm so tired that all I can think about is crawling into bed (alone!).
- My job, plus baby, plus running a household equals very little energy left over for passionate lovemaking. All I want to do at night is sit like a robot in front of the TV and watch reruns.
- My husband doesn't understand me!

## THE NEW FATHER SYNDROME

You may feel that your husband is unaware of or insensitive to the new-mother stresses you have to deal with, but be aware of the changes *he* is going through:

- He's been waiting patiently for the last two months of pregnancy and childbirth for a good night in bed and you tell him you're not in the mood.
- You've been the center of attention for nine months, *now* it's the baby's turn, but when is it *his* turn?
- He's actually jealous of this little thing who seems to be taking all your time. And he feels guilty for feeling jealous.
- He's having trouble accepting his familiar sex partner as the mother of his child.
- He's afraid your sex life is never going to get better—and things will never be good again.

In more extreme cases, reports Dr. Michael E. Murray, professor of psychology at Southern Methodist University, in an article by Ann Rulten in *Sexual Medicine Today* (see Bibliography), an emotionally immature husband may begin seeing another woman or other women during the time when he should be closest to his wife. Most marital situations are not so fragile, but clearly your husband does need special attention—especially now that the baby's here and you *still* can't have sex, or don't feel up to it.

In Latin American countries, the husband is the one celebrated once the baby is born. He is taken out to dinner and hailed for his new role as a father. Except for a clap on the back when he passes out cigars, our society all but neglects the new father. We focus only on the new baby and mother. What can you do to ease your husband through this period?

- Visit your obstetrician together. Have your doctor explain *why* you should abstain from intercourse right after the birth. Have her reassure your husband that his feelings are normal and that this is a period of stress for all couples, no matter how good the marriage.
- Try to get your husband to talk about his feelings—even if he's ashamed of them. Be understanding and sympathetic to his problems.
- Have your husband talk to other new fathers so he can realize that they have many of the same feelings he does.
- Involve your husband in the care of the baby.
- Remind yourself and your husband that you have entered a new phase of your marriage. Now you are both "parenting together." You are a team and the problems of this period will not last forever.
- For you, always remember that your primary relationship is with your husband. Your children grow up and leave, but your husband will always be with you. When things quiet down (and they will!) you will both realize that you love each other as much as always.

## TEN WAYS TO PUT ROMANCE (AND SEX!) BACK INTO YOUR LIFE

1. You have to set priorities in your life. Your husband and sex should be a major priority. If you have to give up keeping the cleanest house in the neighborhood, then do so.
2. Set some small amount of time aside late in the afternoon or when

you get home from the office to comb your hair, put on fresh lip gloss and blusher. Give yourself a spray of your favorite cologne and change into something fresh if necessary.

3. Take advantage of your new nursing figure. Wear something low-cut for a change. Why not? Your full breasts won't last forever.

4. Dr. Gideon Panter says that the first five minutes your husband comes home from work set the mood for the entire evening. Greet your husband lovingly.

5. Use your good dishes even if you're having only hamburgers or Chinese food for dinner. Light a couple of candles and open a bottle of wine.

6. Make a pact with yourself that you will not talk about the baby with your husband for one hour an evening.

7. You sometimes have to plan for sex. If opportunities are not present-ing themselves, then you have to *make* them. Making a date to have sex gives you something to look forward to. If your husband responds poorly to planning, you can secretly set the stage at such a time as after dinner, when the baby's asleep.

8. Buy your husband a sexy little gift (after all, you and the baby have been getting lots of presents). Use your imagination. Give him any-thing from a new bathrobe to a new aftershave lotion. Buying him a man's body moisturizing lotion is a good excuse to give him a body massage.

9. Ask a relative or hire a babysitter to take the baby out for a walk for a couple of hours on a Saturday afternoon. *Stay home.* Spend the time talking, loving, and just getting to know each other again.

10. Take a minivacation without the baby. Leave at twelve noon on Saturday and return twelve noon on Sunday. Express your milk if you're breast-feeding. Stay at a nearby hotel or resort. Have a romantic dinner Saturday evening and sleep late Sunday morning. It will feel as good as two weeks in the sun.

It may require extra effort at first, but working on your sex life is ob-viously most rewarding. It really will help smooth out the postpartum pe-riod for you. After all, sex is most of the reason you put all that effort into your beauty and fitness, what this book is all about.

# CHAPTER·XIV·
# *Coping*

SUSY WAS HAVING A BAD DAY. She forgot the boiling pot of pacifiers until the burning rubber smell brought her racing down the stairs. Her office kept calling while she was either nursing her two-week-old baby or trying to nap. When the baby was finally fed and resting comfortably on her lap, Susy called her frantic coworkers. As they grappled with an office problem over the telephone, she felt something warm and wet on her lap. Sure enough, baby Amanda had a loose bowel movement that leaked through her disposable diaper onto Susy's last clean pair of jeans. When Susy hung up she surprised herself by noisily bursting into tears. "What's happening to me?" she told us she asked herself at the time. "There I sat with greasy hair, oily skin, ten pounds overweight, bleeding lochia, leaking milk, and a smelly baby on my lap. All I could think about was 'What about me?' Everyone's giving all the attention to the baby but what about me? *I'm* the one who needs to be taken care of now."

Susy's one of the reasons we began this book. We felt a book devoted to the pregnant woman and new mother—and *only* to her—was definitely needed. Advertising and TV shows have created a public image of a happy adoring mother and a perfect cooing baby. Did you ever notice how babies on TV *always* stop crying when Mother takes them into another room off-screen? But the reality of new motherhood is far from these blissful scenes.

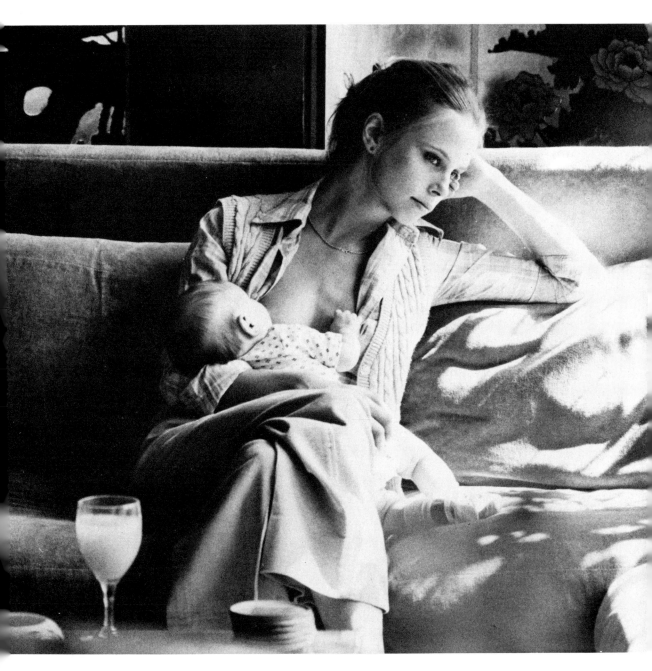

Caring for a new baby can be lonely and exhausting.

There is more anxiety, depression, disappointment, and messed-on jeans than we are led to believe or ever expect. Even when we do hear of post-partum blues and harried moms, many of us first-time mothers secretly believe that we will be more organized than other women, or have "good" babies. But none of us escape some feelings of inadequacy in our new role, as well as twinges of resentment toward the baby for his part in disrupting our life-style. On top of this, we feel conflict between our roles as self-sacrificing mothers and our careers or work outside the home. Expectations imposed by society and personal thinking vie with the reality of having this baby, who makes life change in ways you never believe possible.

With all this happening to you, is it any wonder you sometimes feel that, like Susy, *you*—not the baby—are the one who needs to be taken care of? It's hard under the circumstances to feel good about yourself, to have a pulled-together wardrobe or a crisp new hairdo or a polished and pretty face—and yet spending time on your health, beauty, and energy is as important now as it has ever been in your life. How do you fit it all in? How do you keep from sinking under the weight of your new-mother responsibilities? It *can* be done—you may not believe it at the beginning, but a six-month-old child is easier to care for than a two-week-old and a year-old child is easier to care for than a six-month-old. You will become more organized, get more sleep, be able to think more clearly and have more time to spend on yourself.

## DO ALL NEW MOTHERS FEEL THIS WAY?

If you look and feel depressed and listless after you have your baby, there's a physiological reason for it. Your hormonal system is reverting to its pre-pregnancy state in the time period of six weeks—a reversion that takes its toll on your emotions. The baby needs middle-of-the-night feedings and this interrupted sleep can cause great fatigue. Fatigue, in turn, might trigger a loss of appetite. And, if you are nursing on top of this, you can easily become physically debilitated.

Severe postpartum depression is a matter for your obstetrician or for a psychiatrist, psychologist, or a family counseling service. But what about those of us who just find ourselves crying often, or yelling at our husbands, relatives, and the baby, or feeling frustrated? Don't feel ashamed or guilty—this is normal.

YOU ARE NOT ALONE IF:

- you feel lonely, tired, depressed, exhilarated, scared
- you feel having a baby wasn't such a great idea after all
- you have fantasies about accidentally harming your baby
- you wish you'd had a boy instead of a girl (or a girl instead of a boy)
- you feel you'll scream if one more childless friend asks you, "Well, what did you do all day?"
- you feel you'd like to throttle the next person who offers "helpful" advice
- you feel you're the only one who knows what your baby needs—a babysitter or relative can't really help when the baby's crying
- you stare at your baby in amazement at how miraculous she is
- when you go out to a movie, you haven't the slightest idea of what's going on because you've been thinking of your baby the whole time
- you feel jealous that your husband can leave in the morning to go out to work (and he feels guilty because he's so happy to go!)
- you feel you'll never have the same close relationship with your husband
- you're fascinated and frightened to see a new, warm, almost feminine side of your husband emerge caring for the new baby
- you feel that world news is totally irrelevant—all that matters is your own plight at home with your baby
- you feel you've lost your sense of humor along with your figure
- you feel like you couldn't care less that "the second one is always easier!"

If you feel depressed or simply confused and lonely, try forming a "mother support group"—or join one already in existence. Your prepared-childbirth class is a good source for other mothers looking for such a group. Or, ask your obstetrician (she may report that other mothers are looking for friends too), the hospital (why not your roommate?), the playground, or your pre- or postnatal exercise class. If you don't want something as formal as a mother support group, you can still actively seek out mothers of other young children and share your feelings. Even if you consider yourself a complete, independent woman, there's probably no other time in your life that you'll need other women more for companionship and support.

Quite apart from the hormonal and psychological stresses of new motherhood, you have to cope with a new problem—exhaustion. It drains you of energy and your sense of well-being and plays havoc with your looks: a pale face, red-rimmed eyes, a fatigued posture, are only part of the picture. For the first few months exhaustion can threaten to become a way of life. Don't let it. Doctors believe that the way you treat yourself during this period sets the pace for your recovery in the next nine months, so handle yourself with loving care. Take as much time to rest as you can so that you will start to feel like your old self after six weeks. Some fatigue may be related to anemia, so check with your doctor if you're feeling especially rundown. Simple exhaustion can be combatted with a little planning.

If you didn't learn to nap while you were pregnant, try now. The baby's sleep pattern is sure to wake you up at 2:00 or 4:00 A.M. at the beginning. Even if you get to sleep at 9:30 P.M., interruptions during the night deny the body's need to pass through different stages of deep and lighter sleep. So you must compensate. What can you do to cut down on interruptions?

- Alternate night feedings. *You* nurse or give a bottle one night and *your husband* gives a bottle the next.
- Have your husband get up to change the baby and bring her into your room.
- Stay in bed as long as possible in the morning. Many mothers find that bringing the baby into bed with them in the morning helps prolong their own rest.

- If the baby wakes up in the wee hours, bring him into bed and enjoy this "secret time" with just yourself and the baby. Watch the late late show together, but don't doze off—be aware that rolling over on the baby is a possibility. So if you're a tosser, don't sleep with the baby.

Interrupted sleep isn't the only villain when it comes to fatigue—visiting friends and relatives can wear you down relentlessly, from the kindest of motives. To preserve your equilibrium, use these antidotes for your doting aunts:

- *don't* invite anyone to your house for dinner.
- *do* accept all dinner invitations out.
- be firm about *when and for how long* guests may visit. Have a standard line ready for potential visitors: "I'd love to see you. My doctor is limiting my visitors, but we can spend a half-hour together this afternoon." If guests overstay their welcome, just excuse yourself and go to bed.
- if the telephone's not giving you a moment's peace, take it off the hook, get an answering machine, or install a small device called a silencer, which silences the ringing on your end.
- if your mother, mother-in-law, sister, or a friend has come to help out, let them do just that. They are not company. Don't be afraid to ask them to do things for you. They really do want to help!
- if relatives from out of town are coming in to see the baby, immediately suggest the name of a wonderful hotel where they can stay—not your home. You can play hostess next year!

## SCHEDULING YOUR TIME

Looking and feeling well during the first few months postpartum is, in part, a matter of organization. If you and your household are to function at all efficiently during this time, you will have to schedule and order events in your new life with the baby.

There are three principles to keep in mind here:

ORGANIZE. Since your schedule will revolve around the baby's, many personal and household tasks will have to be done while the baby is asleep. Make lists of what has to be done and when.

DELEGATE AUTHORITY. Share household chores on a prearranged basis with your husband. Consider ordering groceries over the telephone and having them delivered. Try having your linen done by a service.

BREAK THE RULES. There's no law that says you have to make your bed in the morning. Make it when you have time and you feel like it. The same goes for other household chores. Don't feel you have to write or telephone time-consuming thank-you's to people who have sent baby gifts; a pretty postcard with two sentences on it will be fine.

Amid all of this, watch out for yourself. If your lochia turns bright red in the first few weeks at home, or you find yourself so tired you're not eating properly or enjoying the baby, slow down. Solicit help from all available sources and allow yourself to be waited on until you feel strong and energetic.

## GOING BACK TO WORK

"I'm just not the type of person to stay home," said Mike, a fashion buyer for a large department store in New York City. "I knew I wanted to go right back to work after I had Jessica two and a half years ago and I've never had a doubt since. Time I spend with my daughter is good time—time in which we are completely each others', telling stories, playing, taking baths together. I can't really think of anything I don't like about working full-time *and* being a mother."

Mike's uncomplicated attitude, it must be said at the start, is more the exception than the rule. She's had great luck with an excellent and loyal housekeeper. Jessica was a healthy baby who suffered little more than a few sniffles and colds in her little two-and-a-half-year life and Mike's husband is very supportive and helps share the work load at home. Mike loves working and would suffer terribly if she had to give it up—and having two incomes in this newly expanded family doesn't hurt!

When Sheila returned to work two months after Victoria was born, she found herself feeling ambivalent. It was not all that easy to leave the baby in the care of the housekeeper who, she secretly feared, would somehow replace her in her daughter's heart and emotions. When she came home at night and on weekends, she was often so fatigued that she didn't feel she gave Victoria that "quality time" she believed working mothers are supposed to give their children. By the time she got home, Victoria had eaten and was cranky because her bedtime was near.

Sheila was able to work out a solution for her mixed feelings. She found a three-day-a-week job and started taking courses toward her master's. She now has more time with Victoria, but she's not as challenged by her present job and admits she is a little bored.

Most women who return to work do feel some ambivalance. One dedicated corporate lawyer returned to work three months after the birth of her son and worked late evenings as before. "I've had a recurring nightmare. I dream that one day I come home late at night, tiptoe into the nursery and see, not a baby, but a six-year-old boy—I realize I've missed his entire babyhood and growing up. As work oriented as I am, there's obviously some guilt about not staying home with Anthony."

From an age when work and motherhood were thought to be incompatible, we've entered a time when we now have the option to work. In fact, there is often great peer pressure to do so, especially among professional people. It's often hard to make a choice because people have such a bewildering variety of opinions about it. It will help to read and talk with your working friends about any problems you may have.

The elements that seem to be necessary for a comfortable and happy working situation are:

A POSITIVE ATTITUDE. Be proud of your desire to work and secure in the knowledge that it is right for you and your family. If it's necessary to work and you're unhappy about it try going back to school and getting into a field that you find satisfying.

A SUPPORTIVE HUSBAND. He'll have to share the workload and give you emotional support. If he is doubtful or disapproving of your working, try visiting your pediatrician together for a talk.

GOOD CHILDCARE. Make sure that you have the best childcare available.

A FLEXIBLE ATTITUDE TOWARDS YOUR CHILD'S SCHEDULE. If you are absolute about sleeping and eating times, you may have to sacrifice precious time with your baby. Be sensible but don't be rigid.

REALISM. Recognize the fact that you're not superwoman—don't be a perfectionist, or try to be all things to all people.

FLEXIBLE WORK HOURS. If you can, arrange flexible work hours. Take time off for a long lunch visit or an afternoon off with the baby when he is sick. This will help both you and the child.

Remember that children are happy when their parents are happy and your child will love having an interesting and vital father *and* mother. And working does just that—it makes you a parent to be proud of.

## ELECTING TO STAY HOME WITH THE BABY

Women who return to work experience some conflicts and are on call for two major responsibilities. Women who decide to stay home full-time with their first or second baby after working at a job or career or after college may have an equally hard time adjusting. New mothers today have difficulty finding role models, since most of our mothers stayed home and had only one role—that of motherhood. We often have both ultimate career goals and mothering goals. It's hard to combine these two images in our mind, much less in reality. Those who want to stay home feel that a close early bond with the baby is the most important influence in their child's life. But they still cannot help experiencing conflict when they see other women getting out and working. One of our friends made a list of inequities that came with what she called "the strange irony of being a housewife":

- You don't get paid
- You feel like you have to be better at housework because you spend more time at it
- Your role model is that woman in the TV commercial who gets obsessive about "ring around the collar"
- You might have hired cleaning help when you worked, but since you're home you're expected to do all the housework
- Your husband asks you to run all his errands
- You're not contributing to the family expenses—and there are more expenses than ever now
- No one is going to reward you with a raise if your child is the first on the block to learn to read

One of the most frustrating aspects of motherhood, according to Reva Rubin, a psychologist who has studied this postpartum period, is the absence of objective standards to measure success or failure while rearing children.

Mothers who want to stay home with their children at least for a number of years often feel the same kind of pressure from peers or parents as women who choose to go back to work. Try not to feel guilty about your choice. Trust your instinct and enjoy your baby's precious childhood years.

## "WHAT ABOUT ME?"

With all the time and thought you must put into arranging your work and home life, it's easy to forget about taking care of *you*. Don't let that happen. Time spent on yourself is necessary—especially in the first nine months postpartum. One new mother who worked on a national magazine decided to take a few years off with her baby. She found she would pounce on her investment-banker husband when he came home from his office. "What did you do? Who did you talk to? What happened on the stock market? Who's your secretary going out with now?"

"I pelted my husband with a stream of inquiries everyday," she said. "Then I realized I was living through him. There and then I decided I was going to hire a babysitter and have my own interests again. I promptly signed up for two courses—one on folk art and the other on children's literature—at a nearby college. What a difference it made!"

Another woman told us, "I used to get up at six in order to get the baby fed and bathed and the household organized before I got off to work; then I'd be home at five-thirty to make dinner, feed the baby, and put her to bed. After dinner I'd try to catch up on all the office work I'd brought home with me, and I found I was nodding off to sleep over my memos. I needed a haircut and I hadn't bought a new dress (except maternity dresses) in a year—I just didn't have any time for myself!"

Make time for yourself. Whether you're a working mother or stay at home, try to set aside one block of time each day for *you*—whether it's thirty minutes or three hours. Having this to look forward to will go a long way in helping you cope with your new life. This is "selfish sanity" time in which you have a chance to think about anything other than your family. Choose a time such as the baby's naptime, or after the baby is in bed at night. The best solution is to hire a babysitter or other helper who will give you an hour or an afternoon off for reenergizing yourself.

If you've got thirty minutes, give yourself a break:

- Brew a pot of herbal tea. Use your best china cup and saucer and a cloth napkin. Relax in a room other than your kitchen and sip slowly.
- Curl up in bed or on a chaise lounge or a couch with your favorite magazine. Turn the lights very low and put on soft music.
- Call an old friend you haven't spoken to in years and talk about old times—not the babies!

- Look through a photo album of *your* old baby pictures.
- Make a list of gifts *you'd* like to receive for Christmas—even if it's only July.
- Work on a hobby you've always wanted to try—your family's genealogy, crocheting, etc. Choose a hobby that doesn't involve pulling out bunches of supplies that you'll later have to put away.
- Plan a party—even if it's for a year from now!
- Make a list of all the places you would like to go for a vacation.
- Have your newspaper delivered and read it! Many mothers report they can't concentrate for practically nine months, but try to read something light. Reading is an important escape. Try light magazines as well as the paper.
- Buy fresh flowers for yourself.
- Do a special facial relaxing exercise. Many mothers walking past mirrors catch glimpses of themselves frowning or clenching their jaws. You may have to take special care to correct these expressions so they don't become habitual in a tense time like new motherhood. When you feel your jaw tightening up, try this: close your eyes and lean your head back as far as it will go. Let your mouth fall open. Hold this position for the count of ten. Then let your head fall forward and hold for another count of ten. Start rotating your head very, very slowly in one direction. Then rotate in the other direction. Repeat this four times.
- Meditate.

If you've got an afternoon free each week:

- Take a course. Study photography or flower arranging or whatever pleases you.
- Do the volunteer work you've always wanted to do.
- Keep a diary.
- Go shopping.
- Go to an exercise class.
- Play tennis or go for a bike ride.
- Call past business associates and have lunch together. They may have something part-time or freelance for you to do.

Don't forget to do small favors for yourself—buy a new lipstick when you're on your way to the park with the baby, or make a standing lunch date with your best friend. Get other people to start remembering that *you* count, too. If friends and/or relatives want to know what you need as a new mother gift, here are some ideas:

- A casserole, prepared and ready to go in the oven.
- A gift certificate at a salon for a haircut, manicure, pedicure.
- Tickets for you and your husband to a concert.
- Any time-saving device such as a lettuce spinner or a food processor.
- A week's worth of groceries.
- A month's worth of baby supplies, such as formula or disposable diapers.
- If your baby has received his fiftieth stretch suit in the mail and honestly couldn't use another thing until he starts kindergarten, bring it back and use the money on yourself. Don't feel guilty—you deserve it!

P.S. When people come with gifts for the new baby and your older children stand there with sad little faces, be prepared. Have little wrapped five-and-ten-cent gifts on hand so all the children will get things.

## A BEAUTIFUL TIME OF LIFE

It's hard to get perspective when you're in full battle with dirty diapers, little sleep, a chaotic household, and yet another delivery man at the door. But remember that some day you may even be able to laugh at your plight. You need a sense of humor and a sense of history for the first difficult period at home with a new baby. Perhaps most important, you need a firm and positive sense of self. This is a wonderful and beautiful time in your life—your pregnancy and your new motherhood give you a new kind of identity as a woman. We've reminded you to put *you* back in the picture of madonna and child so that you'll awaken to that sense of completeness.

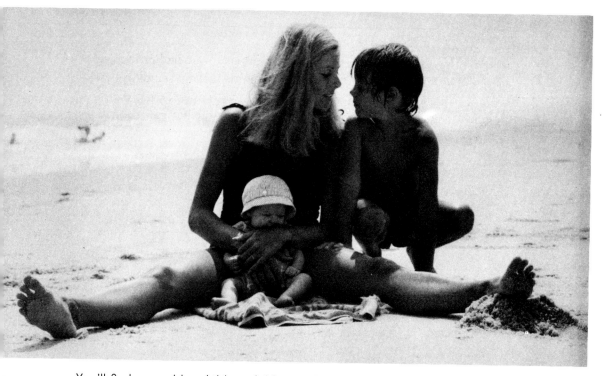

You'll find your older child or children will need extra love and attention when the new baby arrives.

By outlining an eighteen-month beauty program, we've given the specifics for helping you maintain your good looks and good health and achieve new beauty in your role as a pregnant woman and new mother.

We are so lucky to have our babies, now, when being pregnant and carrying on business as usual don't seem incompatible ideas any more. It's all part of the new freedom in childbearing. It is a time to extoll and celebrate *yourself* as a woman—looking pretty, looking your best ever, is now an exciting and well-rewarded goal.

Let pregnancy and motherhood be the prettiest time of your life. In years past having a baby meant letting the event "happen" to us but today we are better informed about all aspects of pregnancy and childbirth. We can take steps to make ourselves pretty, healthy, and energetic these nine months of pregnancy and nine months after. It's up to you.

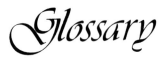

# Glossary

IN THIS BOOK there are medical—especially obstetrical terms—you may be unfamiliar with. This glossary explains these words or terms. Check the index for further references in the text.

AMNIOCENTESIS. A test of the amniotic fluid performed on women who are either over thirty-five, or have a family history of disease, or chromosomal defects to determine whether or not the fetus has chromosomal defects.

ANDROGEN. A hormone that produces masculine characteristics.

ANEMIA. A condition in which blood is deficient in red blood cells, in hemoglobin, or in total volume. It is very often due to an iron deficiency.

AREOLA. The colored area around the nipple.

BREECH BIRTH. A birth in which the baby is born buttocks or feet first.

CAESAREAN SECTION. The delivery of a baby by an operation in which the fetus is removed by making a surgical incision in the wall of the stomach and uterus. See pp. 28–30, 196–97 for more information.

CARCINOGEN. A cancer-producing substance.

CERVIX. The constricted lower end of the uterus that projects into the vagina. The central cervical canal connects the uterine cavity with the vagina.

CHLOASMA (MELASMA or MASK OF PREGNANCY). A hyperpigmentation of the skin characterized by brown or yellow patches on the forehead, cheeks, upper lip, or neck. See pp. 13–15 for more information.

COLLAGEN. The protein contained in connective tissue and bones.

COLOSTRUM. A yellowish sticky fluid secreted by the breasts during pregnancy and for two to three days after delivery. It contains the protein and antibodies a newborn needs.

DERMABRASION (SKIN PLANING). A technique used by doctors to remove scars by abrading the skin with a dermabrasion machine. See pp. 275, 277 for more information.

ECLAMPSIA. An illness of pregnancy marked by convulsions and coma.

EDEMA. Excess fluid retention in the body that may cause swelling. See pp. 120–21 for more information.

ENGORGEMENT. The filling with blood or other fluid to the point of congestion. The genitals often become engorged during pregnancy and the breasts usually become engorged with milk after delivery. See p. 196 for more information on engorgement of the breasts.

EPISIOTOMY. An incision of the tissue between the vagina and the anus allowing more room for the baby to be delivered, thereby preventing possible tearing of the mother's tissues.

ESTROGEN. Any one of a group of female hormones secreted by the ovaries. Estrogen is mainly responsible for female body characteristics and for producing the changes of menstruation and pregnancy.

FETAL MONITOR. Any of a number of devices used to measure the heart rate of the fetus and the strength of maternal contractions.

FETUS. An unborn baby from the third month of development on. (Before that it is usually called an "embryo.")

FORCEPS DELIVERY. A delivery in which forceps are used to grasp the baby's head so that it can be assisted through the birth canal.

GENE. A unit of heredity that determines development of hereditary character.

GERMAN MEASLES (RUBELLA). A disease which, if contracted during pregnancy, can cause birth defects.

GESTATION. The nine-month period of time a woman carries the fetus from conception to delivery.

HEMORRHOIDS. Dilated blood vessels that become bulbous swellings in the anus. See pp. 117–18 for more information.

HERPES SIMPLEX TYPE II. A venereal disease characterized by lesions on the vagina and the surrounding area. See p. 118 for more information.

HORMONES. Compounds secreted by the endocrine glands into the blood, to act at a distant site.

INCONTINENCE. The inability to control urine flow. See pp. 116–17 for more information.

INVOLUTION. The process of the body returning to the nonpregnant state after delivery.

KEGEL EXERCISES. Exercises developed by Dr. Arnold Kegel designed to strengthen the pelvic floor through a series of contractions. See pp. 118–20 for more information.

KERATIN. A protein-like substance found in hair and nails.

LABOR. The process in which the baby emerges from the uterus and descends into the birth canal.

LACTATION. The formulation and/or secretion of milk. Lactation also refers to the period of milk production. Also called *nursing* or *breast-feeding*.

LET-DOWN REFLEX. The bodily mechanism of milk production and ejection determined hormonally and usually stimulated by the infant's sucking the mother's nipple and areola.

LEUKORRHEA. A yellow-white discharge from the vagina during pregnancy. See p. 115 for more information.

LINEA ALBA. The white line running from the naval to the pubic bone. It often becomes pigmented to a brown color during pregnancy and is then referred to as "linea nigra."

LOCHIA. A vaginal discharge that consists of blood from the site in the uterus where the placenta breaks away. See pp. 195, 205–206 for more information.

LOW-BIRTH-WEIGHT BABY. An infant weighting less than about five and a half pounds at birth.

MELANIN. A dark pigment appearing in skin and hair.

MISCARRIAGE. A term for the spontaneous expulsion of the fetus before it is viable.

MULTIPARA. A woman who has had at least one live birth and is pregnant again.

OVARY. The female reproductive gland that produces ova and hormones.

OVULATION. The time during which an egg or ovum is shed from the ovaries. Ovulation occurs approximately every twenty-eight days.

OXYTOCIN. The hormone released during lactation.

PELVIC FLOOR. The floor of muscle layers supporting the pelvic organs. It includes the muscle area starting around the urethra sphincter, continuing to the vagina, and ending at the rectal sphincter.

PERINEUM. The "blank area" extending from the vagina to the rectum.

PFANNENSTEIL (or "BIKINI CUT"). A type of incision used in Caesarean surgery. This incision runs horizontally across the pelvic area. See pp. 28–30 for more information.

PLACENTA. The organ that forms on the lining of the uterus during pregnancy. It provides nourishment and oxygen to the fetus and removes fetal waste products via the umbilical cord. It is also called the "afterbirth" because it is expelled right after delivery.

PLACENTA PREVIA. The condition in which the placenta is abnormally implanted near the cervix as opposed to the fundal portion of the uterus.

POSTPARTUM. The time following childbirth.

POSTPARTUM ALOPECIA. A dermatological term for hair loss after delivery.

POSTPARTUM BLUES (or POSTPARTUM DEPRESSION). Feeling of depression and sadness experienced by some women after having a baby. See pp. 197–98 for more information.

PREGNANCY GINGIVITIS. Inflammation and bleeding of the gums brought on by the hormonal flux of pregnancy. See p. 35 for more information.

PREPARED CHILDBIRTH (or NATURAL CHILDBIRTH). Giving birth with the aids of special breathing and relaxation techniques. Employed during labor and delivery, these techniques eliminate or reduce the need for drugs often administered during childbirth.

"PREPPING." The process by which the nurse "prepares" the woman for delivery. This can include an enema, shaving the perineum, and a vaginal examination.

PROGESTERONE. A hormone that prepares the uterus for the fertilized egg and maintains its development throughout pregnancy.

PUERPERIUM. The period during and just after childbirth.

RELAXIN. A pregnancy hormone that causes joint tissues to relax in order to prepare the body for delivery of the baby.

SEBACEOUS GLANDS. Glands which secrete an oily substance for lubricating hair and skin.

SEBUM. A fatty secretion of the sebaceous or oil glands.

SEMEN (or SEMINAL FLUID). The whitish fluid produced in the male reproductive organs. This fluid contains sperm or spermatazoa responsible for fertilizing the female ovum.

SKIN TAGS. Tiny growths of skin that appear on breasts, areolas, neck, and underarms.

SPIDER VEINS (SPIDER ANGIOMAS or SPIDER NEVAE). Red, spidery marks occuring on the face, neck, and shoulders.

STEROID. A fat-soluble organic chemical. Steroids include sex hormones as well as other compounds.

STRETCH MARKS (STRIAE). Reddish, depressed streaks that can occur on the abdomen, breasts, hips, and buttocks resulting from hormonal changes and stress on the skin. See pp. 11-13 for more information.

TERATOGEN. Drugs, virus, or X rays—exposure to which can cause damage to a fetus.

TESTOSTERONE. Male sex hormone.

TETRACYCLINE. An antibiotic often prescribed for acne.

TOXEMIA (or PREECLAMPSIA). An illness of late pregnancy marked by sudden weight gain, increased blood pressure, and secretion of albumin in the urine. See p. 121 for more information.

TRIMESTER. One of three 3-month periods into which pregnancy is divided.

URETHRA. The canal that carries off the urine from the bladder. In females the urethra is the opening located in front of the vagina.

VAGINA. The canal between the uterus and the vulva.

VARICOSE VEIN. An enlarged or swollen vein that can occur in the legs or near the opening of the vagina. See pp. 106-107 for more information.

VERTICAL CUT. The surgical incision used in a Caesarean section delivery that runs from just below the naval to the pubic bone. See pp. 28-30 for more information.

VULVA. The external female genital organs.

# Bibliography

Beazley, John M., and Bingham, Keith D. "Changes in Hair and Skin Condition during Pregnancy." *The British Journal of Clinical Practice* 27 (November 1973): 425–28.

Bing, Elisabeth. *Moving Through Pregnancy.* Indianapolis/New York: Bobbs-Merrill, 1975.

Bing, Elisabeth, and Colman, Libby. *Making Love During Pregnancy.* New York: Bantam Books, 1977.

The Boston Children's Medical Center. *Pregnancy, Birth and the Newborn Baby.* New York: Delacorte Press/Seymour Lawrence, 1971.

The Boston Women's Health Book Collective. *Our Bodies, Ourselves.* New York: Simon and Schuster, 1971.

Brewer, Gail Sforza, with Brewer, Tom. *What Every Pregnant Woman Should Know.* New York: Random House, 1977.

Chase, Deborah. *The Medically Based No-Nonsense Beauty Book.* New York: Pocket Books, 1976.

Cherry, Sheldon H. *Understanding Pregnancy and Childbirth.* New York: Bantam Books, 1975.

Clausen, Joy Princeton; Flook, Margaret Hemp; and Ford, Boonie. *Maternity Nursing Today.* New York: McGraw-Hill, 1977.

Colman, Arthur D., and Colman, Libby Lee. *Pregnancy: The Psychological Experience.* New York: Bantam Books, 1977.

Committee on Dietary Allowances of the Food and Nutrition Board, National Research Council. *Recommended Dietary Allowances.* Washington, D.C.: National Academy of Sciences, 1974. (Available from: Printing and Publishing Office, National Academy of Sciences, 2101 Constitution Avenue, Washington, D.C. 20418.)

Committee on Maternal Nutrition of the Food and Nutrition Board, National Research Council. *Maternal Nutrition and the Course of Pregnancy.* Washington, D.C.: National Academy of Sciences, 1970. (Available from: Printing and Publishing Office, National Academy of Sciences, 2101 Constitution Avenue, Washington, D.C. 20418.)

Cosmetic, Toiletry and Fragrance Association, Inc. "Update on the Safety Testing of Hair Dyes." July 1977.

The Diagram Group. *Woman's Body.* New York: Paddington Press, 1977.

Dilfer, Carol Stahmann. *Your Baby, Your Body.* New York: Crown Publishers, 1977.

Eiger, Marvin S., and Olds, Sally Wendkos. *The Complete Book of Breastfeeding.* New York: Bantam Books, 1973.

Ferguson, Patricia; Lennox, Thomas; and Lettieri, Dan J., eds. *Drugs and Pregnancy.* Rockville, Md.: National Institute on Drug Abuse, November 1974. (For sale by the Superintendent of Documents, U.S. Government Printing Office, Washington, D.C. 20402. Price $2.70. Stock Number 017-024-00428-6.)

Guttmacher, Alan F. *Pregnancy, Birth and Family Planning.* New York: Signet, 1973.

Habicht, Jean-Pierre; Yarbrough, Charles; Lechtig, Aaron; and Klein, Robert E. "Relation of Maternal Supplementary Feeding During Pregnancy to Birth Weight and Other Sociobiological Factors." *Current Concepts of Nutrition* 2 (1974): 127-45.

Harris, Stephanie G., and Highland, Joseph H. *Birthright Denied: The Risks and Benefits of Breast-feeding.* Environmental Defense Fund, 1977.

Hill, Reba Michels; Craig, Janice P.; Chaney, Margarete D.; Tennyson, Linda M.; and McCulley, Lee B. "Utilization of Over-the-Counter Drugs During Pregnancy." *Clinical Obstetrics and Gynecology* 20 (June 1977): 381-94.

Manzoni, Pablo. *Instant Beauty.* New York: Simon and Schuster, 1978.

Masters, W. H., and Johnson, V. E. *Human Sexual Response.* Boston: Little, Brown and Company, 1966.

Milinaire, Caterine. *Birth*. New York: Harmony Books, 1974.

Miller, Mary Ann, and Brooten, Dorothy A. *The Childbearing Family: A Nursing Perspective*. Boston: Little, Brown and Company, 1977.

Noble, Elizabeth. *Essential Exercises for the Childbearing Year*. Boston: Houghton Mifflin Company, 1976.

Null, Gary, and Null, Stephen L. *Handbook of Skin and Hair*. New York: Pyramid Books, 1976.

Null, Gary; Null, Stephen; and staff. *Successful Pregnancy*. New York: Pyramid Books, 1976.

Panter, Gideon G., and Linde, Shirley Motter. *Now That You've Had Your Baby*. New York: David McKay Company, 1976.

Penney, Alexandra. "Playing Safe With Hair Coloring." *The New York Times Magazine,* February 26, 1978.

Pryor, Karen. *Nursing Your Baby*. New York: Pocket Books, 1973.

Rulten, Ann. "Managing the Sexual Woes of New Fathers." *Sexual Medicine Today* 2 (January 1978): 26–27, 38.

Sims, Naomi. *All About Health and Beauty for the Black Woman*. New York: Doubleday, 1976.

Solberg, Don A.; Butler, Julius; and Wagner, Nathaniel N. "Sexual Behavior in Pregnancy." *The New England Journal of Medicine* 288 (May 24, 1973): 1098–1103.

Tolor, Alexander, and DiGrazia, Paul V. "Sexual Attitudes and Behavior Patterns During and Following Pregnancy." *Archives of Sexual Behavior* 5 (1976): 539–50.

U.S. Department of Health, Education, and Welfare. *Prenatal Care*. Washington, D.C.: Office of Child Development, 1973. (For sale by the Superintendent of Documents, U.S. Government Printing Office, Washington, D.C. 20402. Price 75 cents. Stock Number 1791-00187.)

U.S. Department of Health, Education, and Welfare. *Smoking and Health: A Report of the Surgeon General*. Washington, D.C.: Public Health Service, 1979.

Wilentz, Joel M.; Kantor, Irwin; and Berger, Bernard. "Pregnancy and the Skin." *Cutis*, May 1975, pp. 683–85.

Williams, Phyllis S. *Nourishing Your Unborn Child*. New York: Avon Books, 1975.

Zizmor, Jonathan, and Foreman, John. *Superhair.* New York: G. P. Putnam's Sons, 1978.

Zizmor, Jonathan, and Foreman, John. *Super Skin.* New York: Berkley Medallion Books, 1977.

# Index

Lubricant jelly (or cream), for sex after childbirth, 312, 314, 316
Lubrication, vaginal, 175

Makeover by Pablo Manzoni, 38–43
Makeup, 38–43; chloasma and, 15; five-minute routine, 288–91; for new mothers, 280–84; for stretch marks, 275. *See also specific types of cosmetics*
Malige, Didier, 302
Malnutrition during pregnancy, 72–73
Manzoni, Pablo, 15, 19, 25, 38–43
Marijuana, 251
Mascara, 41
Mask, for dry skin, 24–25; for oily skin, 22–23; yogurt, 284
Massage, for breasts, 113; for dry hair, 53; for feet, 37
Masters, William H., 169, 171, 176–77, 313, 315–16
Masturbating, 182
Maternity clothes, 144–68; accessories, 160–61; adapting your clothes, 147; assembling a new wardrobe, 151–52; bathing suits, 164–65; basic wardrobe checklists, 152, 154; bras, 114, 161–62, 187, 219; conversion to postpartum fashion, 262–63; dresses, 154, 156; girdles, 164; growth stages and, 148–49; outdoor, 167,

168; pants, 158, 160; skirts, 160; slips, 163; stockings, *see* Stockings; tops, 157–58; underpants, 115, 161, 187; where to find, 149, 151
Medications, *see* Drugs
Melanin, 13, 16
Melasma (chloasma), 13–17, 276–78
Menus, 85–87, 89–90
Milk bath, 32
Minerals, 76–78; hair growth and, 300–301. *See also* Vitamin-mineral supplements
Miscarriages, sex and, 176, 177, 183
Moisturizers, 40, 41, 281; after bath, 33; for breasts, 217; for crepey skin, 280; for oily skin, 23; stretch marks and, 13
Moles, 16–17
Montgomery, tubercles of, 112–13
Morning Health Drink, 244
Morning sickness, foods for relieving, 82–83
Mother, reevaluating your relationship with your, 176
Mother support groups, 325–26
Mouth watering, 83
Murray, Michael E., 319–20
Muscles, abdominal, 102, 104–105, 208

Nail polishes, 36, 38
Nails, 35–36, 286–87
Nausea, 79; foods for relieving, 82–83; sex and, 176, 177
Night cream, 25

Nightgowns, 185–86; nursing, 269
Night sweats, 213–214
Nipples, colostrum secreted by, 112, 113; darkening of, 16; exercise for toughening, 114; exposure to air, 113–114; postpartum care of, 216–17
Nursing, *see* Breast-feeding
Nursing pads, 218
Nutrition, *see* Diet

Oily hair, 54–56
Oily skin, 21–24, 279; beauty tips for, 23; cleansing, 21; product checklist for, 24. *See also* Acne; Combination skin
O'Leary, Lydia, 15–16
Oral contraceptives, *see* Birth control pills
Oral sex, 182
Orentreich, Norman, 274, 275, 277, 296
Orgasm, 175, 182, 183
Ouaknine, Pierre, 59, 301
Outdoor wear, 167, 168
Overweight, excuses for being, 254. *See also* Weight gain

Paints, 97, 98
Palms, reddening of the, 18
Panter, Gideon, 30, 32, 317, 321
Panties, 115, 161, 187
Pants, 158, 160, 264
Pantyhose, 18, 163; for varicose veins, 107

# Credits